Epilepsy in Children

Also by Orrin Devinsky, MD

Epilepsy: Patient and Family Guide, Third Edition

Alternative Therapies for Epilepsy (with Steven C. Schachter and Steven V. Pacia)

Epilepsy in Children

What Every Parent Needs to Know

Orrin Devinsky, MD
with Erin Conway, MS, RN, CPNP and Courtney
Schnabel Glick, MS, RD, CDN

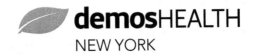

demosHEALTH

NEW YORK

Visit our website at www.demoshealth.com

ISBN: 978-1-936303-78-6
e-book ISBN: 978-1-617052-36-1

Acquisitions Editor: Julia Pastore
Compositor: diacriTech

Medical information provided by Demos Health, in the absence of a visit with a health care professional, must be considered as an educational service only. This book is not designed to replace a physician's independent judgment about the appropriateness or risks of a procedure or therapy for a given patient. Our purpose is to provide you with information that will help you make your own health care decisions.

The information and opinions provided here are believed to be accurate and sound, based on the best judgment available to the authors, editors, and publisher, but readers who fail to consult appropriate health authorities assume the risk of injuries. The publisher is not responsible for errors or omissions. The editors and publisher welcome any reader to report to the publisher any discrepancies or inaccuracies noticed.

Library of Congress Cataloging-in-Publication Data
Devinsky, Orrin, author. | Conway, Erin, author. | Glick, Courtney Schnabel, author.
  Epilepsy in children : what every parent needs to know / Orrin Devinsky, with Erin Conway, and Courtney Schnabel Glick.
  New York, NY : Demos Medical Publishing, LLC, [2016] | Includes bibliographical references and index.
  LCCN 2015038436 | ISBN 9781936303786
  LCSH: Epilepsy in children—Diagnosis. | Epilepsy in children—Treatment. | Epilepsy in children—Diet therapy.
  LCC RJ496.E6 D48 2016 | DDC 618.92/853—dc23 LC record available at http://lccn.loc.gov/2015038436

Special discounts on bulk quantities of Demos Health books are available to corporations, professional associations, pharmaceutical companies, health care organizations, and other qualifying groups. For details, please contact:

Special Sales Department
Demos Medical Publishing, LLC
11 West 42nd Street, 15th Floor
New York, NY 10036
Phone: 800-532-8663 or 212-683-0072
Fax: 212-941-7842
E-mail: specialsales@demosmedical.com

Printed in the United States of America by McNaughton & Gunn.
15 16 17 18 19 / 5 4 3 2 1

*To all of the parents and our patients
who have taught us so much about epilepsy
and even more about caring*

CONTENTS

Preface

The three of us came to health care from very different backgrounds and perspectives—nursing, medicine, and nutrition. Our paths crossed over the care of children with seizures. We have been fortunate to share their lives and learn from them, as well as from their parents and caregivers. This book is inspired by all of our patients and their families. Their questions, experiences, and hope for their child's future are reflected in these pages.

Great questions unfortunately outpace good answers. From diagnosis and treatment options to where the limits of our current knowledge extend, this book will hopefully help parents navigate what at times can be an overwhelming period in their child's life. There has been exponential growth in scientific data, lay Internet sites and community chat rooms, YouTube seizure videos, and disease organizations for which epilepsy is a common thread. The amount of information and connections can be endless and confusing. Our goal is to help parents by providing a home base in the pages of this book to better understand seizures and epilepsy.

We hope to simplify the information while keeping the depth and extent of coverage sufficient to make it comprehensible, approachable, and informative. There is a wide range of the epilepsies in childhood. Seizure types in infants can differ greatly from those in toddlers. Parents should understand their child's epilepsy, but understanding it in the context of the spectrum of epilepsy and associated disorders can better place their child's disorder in perspective.

There is no single face of pediatric epilepsy. Many children with epilepsy enjoy extremely successful academic, social, and athletic lives. Others face challenges—ranging from mild attention and learning disorders to severe limitations in communication, psychiatric disorders, and physical limitations. This diversity presented our greatest challenge. There is a desire to paint the world through rose-colored glasses so as to help overshadow, at least in part, the stigma that has long cast a dark shadow on these children. Parents have the greatest power to disarm stigma through understanding and comfort. They must first come to accept epilepsy—what it means and doesn't mean. It is important to see through the epilepsy and other disabilities and see their children for who they are. The truth is more simple and enduring. We strove to follow our own advice.

Parents have assumed a new role in health care. They have transitioned from passive passengers on a journey led by the health care team into active participants. Indeed, parents have fueled much of the innovation in epilepsy research, access to information, advocacy, and how health care is delivered. Parents not only challenge us to do more, they help us provide more sensitive care, think of more ambitious research questions, collaborate in novel ways, and to join forces as partners. We hope this book empowers more parents to challenge and encourage all health care providers to work together in the fight against epilepsy.

Acknowledgments

All ventures are collaborations, and this one extends far beyond the three authors. We hope to have accurately and accessibly conveyed a snapshot of our medical knowledge and quality-of-life issues for children with epilepsy. While these pages largely reflect our perspective, we knew that our view was too constrained and occasionally flawed. We leaned on our colleagues and our patients' parents to keep us honest. They reminded us when our views were contradicted by facts and when our answers failed to capture the nuances or diversity of reality. We cannot thank them enough: Peter Camfield, Karina Fischer, Jacqueline French, Mike Jasulavic, Warren Lammert, Eric Marsh, Kate Pico, Angela Stone, and Maggie Varadhan.

We are also deeply indebted to Leigh Ann Hirschberg and Julia Pastore, who provided invaluable editorial input to this effort.

UNDERSTANDING EPILEPSY

All forms of seizures are caused by an excessive release of electrical activity in the brain. But what these seizures look like, and how they affect the life of the child in whom they appear, can vary greatly. Epilepsy is a disorder with a tendency toward two or more seizures.

WHAT IS EPILEPSY? AN OVERVIEW

Epilepsy is any condition in which a person has seizures that persist over time. There are many types (syndromes) of epilepsy and many types of seizures. These types of epilepsy vary in their symptoms and causes, though often the cause is unknown. One thing all epilepsies have in common is that they affect the brain and feature seizures as a main symptom. In fact, the word epilepsy comes from the Greek word *epilambanem*, meaning "to seize."

What exactly is a seizure? A seizure is a brief, excessive discharge of electrical activity in the brain that changes how a person feels, senses, thinks, or behaves. When your brain is functioning normally, the stimulation (excitation) of its cells and the dampening (inhibition) of that stimulation are in balance. Epileptic seizures happen when an abnormality in the brain's coordination and control of this nerve-cell activity disrupts the balance. Some seizures are quite minor and might go completely unnoticed by a patient or parent. Others are unmistakable. Some seizures don't require any treatment, and some respond easily and completely to treatment and will have little impact on a child's quality of life. Other seizures require extensive treatment and/or may not respond well to treatment. We go into specific types of seizures in Chapter 2 and specific types of epilepsy syndromes in Chapter 3. (For more about the brain's anatomy and how it functions, turn to Appendix A.)

TERMS AND TOOLS

As you begin learning about your child's particular type of seizures and syndrome, you'll encounter diagnostic and treatment tools mentioned later in this book. One of the most common diagnostic tools, and most frequently referenced in these pages, is an *electroencephalogram*, commonly known as an EEG. An EEG reading is taken by a machine that measures the electrical activity in a person's brain using flat disks temporarily attached to the person's scalp. It is a painless test, but does not always provide diagnostic information. (For more about the EEG, see Chapter 5.) For example, some people with epilepsy have normal EEG results, the same as a person without epilepsy. Others show the characteristic *spike-and-wave* pattern that can definitively diagnose certain epilepsy syndromes. This illustrates one of the most important truths about epilepsy: every case is different, as every child is different, and a test or treatment that works for many patients may not show results in your particular child. This is why diagnosis and treatment for the disorder can involve quite a bit of trial and error. That's not a failing on your medical team's part, but merely a fact when dealing with epilepsy. Diagnosis is often complicated. Sometimes it turns out that your child's seizures are actually not epilepsy. Some patients are revealed not only to have epilepsy, but to have more than one type of seizure or syndrome. And finally, these things can change over time. A child with one type of seizure when diagnosed can develop a second type of seizure or syndrome, or may find that the seizures disappear altogether. All of these are reasons that open, comfortable communication between parents and their child's health care team is vital, as is an understanding that there won't always be quick or easy answers.

We'll also talk a lot about *antiepileptic drugs (AEDs)*, since they're the first line of treatment for many children. AEDs are drugs that have been specifically approved for the treatment of epilepsy and have proven successful for certain syndromes and seizures. The idea of their child going on drugs can seem scary at first for some parents, but the proliferation of AEDs is good news. These medications have helped to control seizures and have brought a better quality of life to many children. The same can be said about surgery and the dietary therapies and medical devices now being used to treat epilepsy. When we talk about *dietary therapies*, we're referring to the ketogenic and related diets that require careful monitoring of your child's meals but have shown great success in lessening seizures. Any treatment that your doctor recommends will be one that's almost certainly deemed safe and likely to help your child. Whatever the course your child's epilepsy takes, your child's well-being should remain the central concern with each decision you and the medical team make. This means that your decisions will be based not simply on whether the treatment works to stop the seizures, but also on its side effects and how the treatment will affect your child's quality of life. Managing epilepsy is a matter of finding this appropriate balance between treatment, side effects, and quality of life. Sometimes finding that balance is easy, but sometimes it means making compromises.

LOOKING AHEAD

It can help to think of epilepsy simply as a seizure disorder, which to many people sounds less frightening than the word *epilepsy* itself. Try to remember that the disorder is only one facet of your child's life, even though at times it can feel all-encompassing. And as seizures can be outgrown, so can epilepsy: 70 percent of children with epilepsy outgrow the disorder.

Even before outgrowing their seizures, most children with epilepsy live normal or near-normal lives. Approximately 50 million people worldwide have epilepsy, and the majority are able to work or go to school and have full academic, athletic, and social lives. Still, some children do have more severe cases of epilepsy, more complicated syndromes, more demanding treatment plans, or cases that don't respond to treatment. Many of these epilepsies are accompanied by intellectual disabilities, autism, depression, anxiety, and physical disabilities. We have written this book to help *all* children with epilepsy, whether their disorder is merely a bump in the road or whether it paves a more difficult path. Our understanding of brain function remains very limited, but is growing exponentially, and many new therapies are being developed. In the meantime, understanding your child's own seizures and syndrome is the first step in confirming a diagnosis and working toward effective treatment.

2 | WHAT KIND OF SEIZURE IS IT? A GUIDE

The first sign that your child has epilepsy will usually be a seizure. But what this seizure looks like—its specific features, how it presents itself—depends on what kind of seizure your child has experienced. This is because seizures vary greatly. Some involve obvious muscle jerks or an unmistakable stiffening of the muscles, while other common types of seizures mimic everyday behavior (such as simple staring) and are easy for a parent or onlooker to miss. In this chapter we'll look in detail at the types of seizures children experience. In the following chapter we'll go one step further to see how identifying and understanding your child's seizure type can help determine her prognosis and treatment.

Overall, epileptic seizures fall broadly into two groups: generalized seizures and focal (also called partial) seizures (Table 2.1). Generalized seizures begin with widespread, excessive electrical discharge that involves both sides of the brain at the same time. In contrast, focal seizures start in a more limited area of the brain. Determining whether your child has generalized or focal seizures is critical because the diagnostic tests and the drugs used to treat generalized seizures differ from those used to treat focal seizures. In diagnosing the seizures, your doctor will ask you (and your child, if old enough) for descriptions of what happened before, during, and after the episode. The doctor will also look at recordings of the electrical activity generated by the child's brain (known as *brain waves*) on an electroencephalography (EEG) scan. With generalized seizures, the EEG shows a widespread increase in electrical activity over both sides of the brain at the same time. In focal seizures, the test shows a more restricted, or local, increase. Focal epilepsy waves can arise independently from either side of the brain, and while they may be more widely distributed over one side, they can appear in both. Yet unlike generalized epilepsy waves, focal waves do not arise simultaneously from both sides of the brain.

EEG results aren't always enough on their own or with your child's history to determine which type of seizures are being experienced, particularly because an EEG can be normal in people with epilepsy and it can show spikes

TABLE 2.1: CLASSIFICATION OF EPILEPTIC SEIZURES

Generalized Seizures

Tonic–clonic

Absence
    Typical
    Atypical
    With special features
        Myoclonic absence
        Eyelid myoclonia

Myoclonic

Clonic

Atonic

Tonic

Focal (Partial) Seizures (Seizures Originating in Specific Parts of the Brain)

Simple partial seizures (consciousness not impaired)
    With motor symptoms (jerking, stiffening)
    With somatosensory (touch) or specialized sensory (smell, hearing, taste, sight) symptoms
    With autonomic symptoms (heart rate change, internal sensations)
    With psychic symptoms (déja vu, dreamy state)
Complex partial seizures (consciousness impaired, automatisms usually present)
    Beginning as simple partial seizures
    Beginning with impairment of consciousness
Partial seizures secondarily generalized to tonic–clonic seizures

in people who have never had a seizure. As a result, doctors may look at hereditary factors, which can play a role in all types of epilepsy but are more common when the seizures are generalized. Even then, it can be tough to make a firm diagnosis. For example, certain seizures (tonic–clonic/grand mal, discussed in the next section) can begin as generalized seizures or as partial seizures. Similarly, a staring spell can be a symptom of an absence seizure (a type of generalized seizure), of a complex partial seizure (a focal seizure, see "Types of Focal (Partial) Seizures"), or a lapse of attention unrelated to epilepsy. One way that you, as a parent, can help the medical team classify seizures is by noting your child's level of consciousness during her episodes. Recording a video of the seizure or possible seizure can be very helpful.

CONSCIOUSNESS DURING SEIZURES: A KEY TO DIAGNOSIS

If you or someone else witnesses your child during a seizure, it's helpful to note or try to remember afterwards how alert and responsive—in other words, how conscious—the child was during this time. Knowing whether your child remained fully conscious, whether her consciousness was impaired, or if her consciousness was lost during the seizure helps classify the seizure type and allows the doctor to make recommendations about what activities are safe for your child to pursue.

To a neurologist, *consciousness* is a person's ability to respond and to remember. People with some kinds of seizures do not recall the seizures afterwards, sometimes remaining totally unaware that they've even had a seizure. Others are aware that they've had a seizure, but are convinced that they didn't experience any loss or impairment of consciousness when, in fact, they did. Therefore, it's helpful, if possible, for you or another witness to test your child during a seizure by asking her to follow commands such as "show me your left hand" and "remember the word yellow." If she can follow the command and remember the word, you can conclude that consciousness was preserved, at least during the time tested.

While neurologists describe consciousness during seizures as either "impaired" or "preserved," the line between these categories is often blurred. Some patients report being "half conscious, present but absorbed in my thoughts," for example. Consciousness can also be considered affected if your child's responsiveness isn't altered but her memory is impaired during an attack. For example, she may be able to respond well during a seizure and perform complex tasks, but later will be unable to recall some details of the episode. Other seizures may impair a child's ability to move voluntarily. This child will be unable to speak or raise her hand when asked but may still be able to recall the entire event afterwards. In this example, consciousness is considered preserved; however, motor control was impaired. Note how long the impairment of consciousness lasts and if it is followed by tiredness.

TYPES OF GENERALIZED SEIZURES

Generalized seizures take a number of forms, as you'll read in this section, but all have one thing in common: they begin simultaneously from both sides of the brain. The common types of generalized seizures are absence seizures, atypical absence seizures, atonic seizures, myoclonic seizures, tonic seizures, and tonic–clonic seizures. They're described here in roughly alphabetical order.

Absence Seizures

Seven-year-old Frank often "blanks out" for a few seconds, sometimes for as long as 10 to 20 seconds. His teacher calls his name, but he doesn't seem to hear her. He usually blinks repetitively, and with the longer seizures his eyes may roll up a bit. With the short seizures he merely stares. Then he is right back where he left off. Some days he has more than 50 of these spells. ■ ■ ■

Absence seizures are marked by brief episodes of staring, during which a person's awareness and responsiveness are impaired. (Absence seizures have historically been called *petit mal,* but doctors do not use this term any more.) The episodes usually last less than 10 seconds, but can last as long as 20 seconds or (infrequently) longer. The seizures begin and end suddenly. There is no warning before the seizure, and immediately afterwards the person is again alert and attentive and often unaware that a seizure has taken place. Typical absence seizures appear simply as "stares," but some absence seizures also feature muscle jerks in the face, shoulders, or eyelids. In other absence seizures, often those lasting more than 10 seconds, the staring is accompanied by changes in muscle activity that can include slight tasting movements of the mouth or rubbing the fingers together.

These spells commonly begin when a child is between ages 4 and 14. In approximately 75 percent of these children, absence seizures will not continue after age 18. Often, absence seizures can be brought on by rapid breathing (hyperventilation), and they usually can be reproduced using this technique in the doctor's office if the patient is not taking medication. The good news for active children is that rapid breathing during exercise doesn't tend to bring on these seizures. Children with absence seizures usually have normal development and intelligence, but they may have higher rates of behavioral, educational, and social problems than other children.

An EEG is extremely helpful in diagnosing absence seizures. In most cases, the EEG taken during an absence seizure will show characteristic generalized spike-and-wave discharges at three to four per second, especially during hyperventilation (see Chapter 5, Figure 5.3). Neuroimaging tests such as an MRI (see Chapter 5) aren't needed in these cases, since MRIs show normal results in children with absence seizures.

Absence seizures can be confused with certain focal seizures such as complex partial seizures (discussed later in this chapter), though absence seizures are usually briefer (less than 20 seconds) and are not associated with a warning (aura) or post-episode symptoms such as tiredness.

Atypical Absence Seizures

It is hard for Kathy's mother to tell when Kathy is having one of her staring spells. During the spells, she doesn't respond as quickly as at other times. The problem is that she is often inattentive, and even when I watch the seizure on the video EEG, it is hard for me to clearly recognize them. ■ ■ ■

The staring spells that indicate *atypical absence seizures* usually begin before a child is six years old. In contrast with typical absence seizures, atypical absence seizures tend to start and end gradually (over seconds), often last more than 10 seconds (their usual duration is 5–30 seconds), and aren't usually provoked by rapid breathing. During these seizures, the child stares but often experiences only a partial reduction in responsiveness. Eye blinking or slight jerking movements of the lips may occur. The children affected by these seizures often have cognitive challenges and are also prone to having seizures of other types (myoclonic, tonic, and tonic–clonic). Atypical absence seizures can be hard to distinguish from the child's usual behavior, especially in children with lower intelligence.

Most children who experience these seizures will have an abnormal EEG, showing slow spike-and-wave discharges, even when a seizure is not currently happening. Atypical absence seizures often continue into later childhood.

Atonic Seizures

Bob's "drop" seizures are his biggest problem. During these seizures, he falls to the ground and often hits his head and bruises his body. Even if someone is right next to him and prepared, they may not catch him. As for protection, we used a helmet for a while but stopped because it didn't prevent injuries and it annoyed him. ■ ■ ■

In an *atonic seizure*, the person suddenly loses muscle strength. Her eyelids may droop, her head may nod, she may drop objects that she's holding, and she may fall to the ground. Atonic seizures usually begin in childhood. Although they last less than 15 seconds, they frequently cause sudden falls that result in injury. When patients with "drop seizures" are studied carefully, sometimes it turns out that they actually have *tonic* seizures (associated with muscle contraction, see "Tonic Seizures" section in this chapter) and not *atonic* seizures.

Clonic Seizures

Susie's seizures start suddenly with these jerking movements of her face or arms. Sometimes the jerks are very visible, other times they are really subtle and after she tells me, I have to look carefully to see them. The seizures tend to be brief, but on occasion, they have gone on for more a minute. ■ ■ ■

Clonic seizures are relatively uncommon and are defined by rhythmic jerking movements of the face, arms, and/or legs. These seizures cause jerking (clonic) movements on both sides of the face and/or limbs but without the stiffening (tonic) component seen in the more common tonic–clonic seizures. In children with juvenile myoclonic epilepsy, some tonic–clonic seizures are preceded by jerking movements (clonic–tonic–clonic seizures). In isolation, clonic seizures are not followed by a prolonged period of confusion or tiredness.

Myoclonic Seizures

In the morning Susie gets the "jumps." Her arms just fly up for a second. She may spill her milk or drop a pen. Sometimes she gets a few of these jumps in a row. After she's had a friend sleep over and is exhausted, the jumps are much more common. ■ ■ ■

Myoclonic seizures appear as brief, shock-like jerks of a muscle or group of muscles. They sometimes occur in people who do not have epilepsy. For example, have you ever fallen asleep and felt your body suddenly jerk? You've experienced *sleep jerks* or *benign sleep myoclonus*. Abnormal forms of myoclonus can be either epileptic or nonepileptic.

Epileptic myoclonus usually causes abnormal movements on both sides of the body at the same time and involves the neck, shoulders, upper arms, body, and upper legs. Some patients describe the seizure as feeling like a "shiver" or "electricity." This seizure type is often part of a syndrome that can usually be well controlled, but in rare cases it may be part of a more serious condition (see Chapter 3).

Tonic Seizures

Jeff just stiffens up. Both of his arms are raised over his head and he grimaces, as if someone is pulling on his cheeks. If he is standing, he may lose his balance and fall. The episode lasts about 10 seconds and he recovers quickly, though if he has a few of these seizures close together, he'll often end up feeling tired. ■ ■ ■

Tonic seizures usually last less than 20 seconds and are associated with sudden stiffening movements of the body, arms, or legs that involve both sides of the body. They are more common during sleep or when a person is in the transition into or out of sleep. If the seizure occurs while a person is standing, she'll often fall. Tonic seizures are most common in children who have cognitive challenges, but they can occur in any child or adult.

Tonic–Clonic (Grand Mal) Seizures

Heather's seizures last only a minute, but to her mother seem as if they last an eternity. This is why they frighten her mother. She can often tell they're coming because Heather becomes crankier than usual and out of sorts. Heather then shrieks with an unnatural cry, falls, and every muscle in her body tenses. Her teeth clench. Even though her mother knows Heather can't swallow her tongue, she still worries that her daughter will. Shortly after the seizure begins, Heather's arms and upper body start to jerk while her legs remain more or less stiff. This is the longest part. Then it finally stops and Heather is out cold. ■ ■ ■

Tonic–clonic (grand mal) seizures are convulsive seizures. The person briefly stiffens (tonic phase) and loses consciousness, falls, and often utters a cry. It is not a cry from pain, but from air being forced through contracting vocal cords. This tonic phase is followed by jerking (clonic phase) of the arms and legs. The seizure usually lasts from one to three minutes. During this time, excessive saliva may be produced, resulting in an effect that's sometimes described as "foaming at the mouth." If the person bites her tongue or cheek, bleeding can result. Loss of urine or, rarely, a bowel movement may occur. Afterwards, the person is tired and confused for a period of time that can last minutes or hours, and often she goes to sleep, though she may end up agitated or depressed. The time immediately after the seizure is called the *postictal* period. (First aid related to these seizures is discussed in Chapter 5, as well as in Appendix B.)

When a person experiences tonic–clonic seizures lasting more than 10 minutes (some define it as longer than five minutes) or recurring in a series of three or more episodes between which the person doesn't return to a normal state, it's called *convulsive status epilepticus*. This condition is dangerous and requires medical treatment, such as rectal diazepam or nasal midazolam (see Chapter 10). The exact duration of continuous seizure activity that is harmful to the brain is not well defined, however, and children appear to tolerate seizures longer than five minutes better than adults do.

TYPES OF FOCAL (PARTIAL) SEIZURES

Focal seizures are set off by an abnormal burst of electrical activity in a restricted area of the brain. Most focal seizures arise from the brain's temporal or frontal lobes. Cortical malformations, head injury, brain infections, stroke, and brain tumors can cause these seizures. In some cases, hereditary factors also play a role. In many cases, no cause can be identified.

Partial (focal) seizures are traditionally divided into three main types. The first distinction rests on whether the patient's consciousness remains fully preserved during the episode. *Simple partial seizures* occur when the patient remains alert, able to respond to questions or commands, and can remember what has happened. If the person's ability to pay attention or to respond to questions or commands is impaired to some degree, a *complex partial seizure* has taken place. Often, a person retains no memory of what happened during all or part of a complex partial seizure. The distinction between simple and complex partial seizures is critical, because the ability to drive, operate dangerous equipment, swim alone, and perform other activities usually has to be restricted in people with uncontrolled complex partial seizures. The third type of partial seizure is one that spreads widely to become a *secondarily generalized tonic–clonic (grand mal) seizure*.

A newer classification scheme being used by some doctors describes focal seizures by their specific features. In this system, a focal seizure is described as having autonomic (the autonomic nervous system regulates key automatic processes like heart rate and breathing), motor, sensory, or other characteristics. Notably, in this scheme *dyscognitive focal seizures* roughly correspond to *complex partial (focal) seizures*.

Simple Partial Seizures

Thomas senses a funky burnt smell and then gets a sense of déja vu, as if he has lived through this moment before and he even knows what is going to be said next. ■ ■ ■

A pressure begins in Rachel's stomach and rises up to her chest, and she gets a sense of anxiety or fear. Sometimes this is all that happens, but other times she goes on to have a tonic–clonic seizure. ▪ ▪ ▪

Simple partial seizures can cause a remarkably diverse array of symptoms. In some cases, the symptoms are not recognized as a seizure, since they can also be explained by other factors. For example, when a person experiences abdominal discomfort it's usually because of a gastrointestinal disorder, but it can also be a symptom of a partial seizure. A tingling sensation in the little finger that spreads to the person's forearm can result from a seizure, but it could also be caused by a migraine or a nerve disorder (such as a"pinched nerve"). The main categories of simple partial seizures are motor, sensory, autonomic, and psychic.

Simple partial seizures that are *motor seizures* affect muscle activity. Most often, the body stiffens or muscles begin to jerk in one area of the body, such as a finger or the wrist. These abnormal movements may remain restricted to one body part, or they may spread to involve other muscles on the same side or both sides of the body. Some partial motor seizures cause localized muscle weakness that can also impair speech. Motor seizures can also produce coordinated actions such as laughter or automatic hand movements.

Sensory seizures cause changes related to sensation. Most often, a person experiencing this type of simple partial seizure has a hallucination—the sensation of something that is not there, such as a feeling of"pins and needles"in a finger, tasting"bitter"on her tongue, or seeing a colored pinwheel. These abnormal sensations may remain restricted to one area or may spread. The person may also sense an illusion, a distortion of a true sensation. For example, a parked car appears to be moving, or a person's voice sounds muffled. These kinds of hallucinations and illusions can involve any of the senses, including touch (numbness, tingling), smell (often an unpleasant odor), taste, vision (a spot of light, a scene with people), and hearing (a click or ringing, a person's voice), as well as vestibular sensations (a floating or spinning feeling).

Autonomic seizures cause automatically controlled bodily functions, such as heart rate or sweating, to change. The human emotion (limbic) system is closely connected to the autonomic nervous system. This is why strong emotions such as fear are associated with increases in the heart rate and breathing rate, sweating, and a sinking feeling in the chest. Partial seizures commonly arise from the limbic areas, and therefore, autonomic changes are common during partial seizures. During an autonomic partial seizure, a person will often experience a strange or unpleasant sensation in her abdomen, chest, or head; changes in her heart rate or breathing rate; sweating; or goose bumps that arise for no reason.

Psychic (dyscognitive) seizures affect how a person thinks, feels, and experiences things. These seizures can impair language function, causing garbled speech, an inability to find the right word, or difficulty understanding spoken or written language, as well as problems with time perception and memory. Psychic seizures sometimes bring on sudden and often intense emotions such as fear, anxiety, depression, or happiness. Unlike normal emotions that are triggered by an external event or internal thought, psychic seizures provoke spontaneous emotions that "come out of the blue." Other feelings associated with psychic seizures are the sense that a person experienced or lived through this moment before (*déja vu*), the sense that familiar things are strange and foreign (*jamais vu*), the feeling that one is not oneself (depersonalization), that the world is not real (derealization), or that one is in a dream or watching oneself in a movie or from outside one's own body.

Complex Partial Seizures

Harold's spells begin with a warning: he says he is going to have a seizure and usually sits down. When asked what he feels, he either doesn't answer or just says, "I feel it." He makes a funny face, as if in mild distress. He then simply stares. He may look when his name is called, but he never answers. During this part, he may make tasting movements with his lips. If he is sitting, he often grabs the arm of the chair and squeezes it. Other times, he touches his shirt, as if picking lint off it, even though it's clean. This lasts a minute or two, and as he comes back he asks questions. He never remembers what he asks or says during these moments directly following the seizure. He is tired afterwards; if he has two of these episodes in the same day, he goes to sleep after the second one. ▪ ▪ ▪

Susan's seizures usually occur when she's asleep. She makes a grunting sound, as if she is clearing her throat. She sits up in bed, opens her eyes, and stares. She may clasp her hands together. When asked if she's OK, she doesn't say a word. Within a minute, she lies back down and goes back to sleep. ▪ ▪ ▪

During *complex partial seizures* (*psychomotor or temporal seizures*), consciousness is impaired but not lost. The person typically stares but cannot respond to questions or commands. If she does respond, she does so incompletely and inaccurately. Automatic movements (*automatisms*) occur in many complex partial seizures. Automatisms can involve the mouth and face (lip smacking, chewing, tasting, and swallowing movements), the hands and arms (fumbling, picking, tapping, or clasping movements), vocalizations (grunts, repetition of words or phrases), or more complex acts (walking or mixing foods in a bowl). Less common automatisms include laughing*, screaming, crying, running, shouting, bizarre and sometimes sexual-appearing movements, and disrobing. Complex partial seizures usually last between 20 seconds and 3 minutes. Auras (simple partial seizures) commonly occur in the seconds before complex partial seizures

---

* Seizures that include laughing automatisms are referred to as gelastic seizures. They can occur with partial seizures arising from temporal or frontal lobes, or from lesions such as a benign tumor affecting the hypothalamus. Patients with hypothalamic lesions and gelastic seizures may experience puberty at an early age and exhibit aggressive behavior.

alter a person's consciousness. After the seizure, a person often feels lethargic or confused, though usually for less than 15 minutes. Complex partial seizures occur in people of all ages.

Some people are unaware that they have had a complex partial seizure. Many of the symptoms are so subtle that from the outside it simply looks as if the person is "thinking about something," "daydreaming," or "spacing out." These episodes usually cause memory lapses. It's possible for a person to perform complex activities during these seizures and then to have no recollection of them afterwards. One doctor undergoing this type of seizure found himself in his hospital's lobby and realized that he was supposed to examine a patient. He went to see the patient, and he examined her. To his amazement, when he went to write up his examination, he found that he had just been to see the patient and already correctly diagnosed pneumonia. He had no recollection of this first examination. He had probably examined her and made his notes right before he had a complex partial seizure, which erased his memory for a short period.

Automatisms can sometimes cause embarrassment and other problems when they result in, for example, a child getting up during class and mumbling or touching the arm of another child. Embarrassing automatisms are fortunately uncommon and, by educating teachers and others who are with the child, their negative consequences can be greatly diminished.

Secondarily Generalized Seizures

This seizure starts with a tingling in Madeleine's right thumb. Then her thumb starts jerking. Within a few seconds, her entire right hand is jerking. She has learned to start rubbing and scratching her forearm, since sometimes she can stop the seizure this way. Other times the jerking spreads up her arm. When it reaches the shoulder, she passes out and her whole body shakes. ■ ■ ■

William sees a colored ball on his right side. The ball grows and fills up his whole view. As the ball grows, everything becomes like a dream, and he doesn't feel real. He says it's the strangest feeling. The seizure may just stop and his vision is just a little blurry—or it can go all the way, causing him to fall to the floor and have a tonic–clonic seizure. ■ ■ ■

When a partial seizure's discharge starts in a localized area but spreads to involve both sides of the brain, it may be a case of a partial seizure evolving into a tonic–clonic seizure. Partial seizures evolve into tonic–clonic seizures in more than 30 percent of children and adults with focal epilepsy. When it happens, it's called a *secondarily generalized seizure*. Patients experiencing this type of evolving seizure may or may not recall having had an aura, and witnesses to these seizures may first observe a complex partial seizure that progresses to a tonic–clonic seizure. This type of tonic–clonic seizure can be difficult to distinguish from a generalized tonic–clonic seizure (as occurs in a generalized epilepsy), especially if no one witnesses it or if it occurs during sleep. However, most convulsive seizures in sleep begin as partial seizures. An EEG and MRI may help distinguish these seizure types.

AFTER THE SEIZURE: WHAT TO LOOK FOR

Knowing what happens in the moments directly after a seizure, referred to as the postictal period, can also help your child's doctor diagnose any seizures. For example, absence seizures are not followed by any postictal symptoms—when the seizure ends, the child's activity resumes as if nothing had happened. After complex partial seizures, however, a child will tend to be slightly confused and tired, usually for less than 5 to 15 minutes. Immediately after a tonic–clonic seizure, the child appears limp and unresponsive, and may be pale or bluish (cyanotic). On awakening, the child often complains of muscle soreness and headache, and of pain in the tongue or cheek if those areas were bitten. The child may be confused and tired, and may sleep. Other postictal symptoms can include impairments in vision, touch sensation, language, and other functions. Try to carefully observe your child after seizures, and be sure to report any postictal behavior to her doctor.

In addition to helping determine the type of seizure your child has experienced, the nature of postictal problems can help identify the area where the seizure began. For example, weakness in the right arm and leg may follow a seizure that began in or near the motor area of the brain's left hemisphere. These postictal symptoms often improve after minutes or hours, but they can also be more prolonged. Weakness of an arm or leg after a focal motor or tonic–clonic seizure may indicate a condition known as Todd's paralysis, which usually resolves over minutes to hours.

For some patients, postictal symptoms such as fatigue, depression, confusion, memory impairment, or headache can be more troublesome than the seizure itself. In some cases simply changing the child's seizure medication may alleviate these symptoms. In other cases, additional medications for specific symptoms, such as headaches, may be helpful.

WHEN SEIZURE PATTERNS CHANGE

Many people with epilepsy experience more than one type of seizure. For example, a child may have both simple and complex partial seizures; or absence, myoclonic, and tonic–clonic seizures. In addition, the features of each type of seizure may change from seizure to seizure or, more often, the features may evolve over months and years. The features of simple partial seizures that precede a person's tonic–clonic episodes are usually consistent, but may change, for example, from experiencing an unpleasant smell and a strange stomach sensation to simply feeling a sensation of chest discomfort. Or a child who'd previously experienced a warning before seizures may no longer have any warning.

These alterations in a person's seizures may result from changes in the spread pattern of the electrical discharge that led to the seizure in the first place. In the case of a child whose aura (simple partial seizure) no longer precedes a tonic–clonic seizure, the area from which the seizure begins and the intensity of the discharge probably have not changed, but the electrical activity may now be taking different pathways that allow it to spread more rapidly. In this instance, the absence of a warning may prevent the child from avoiding injury even though the seizure is no more severe than before.

Children with mild seizures, such as simple partial or absence seizures, later may begin experiencing tonic–clonic seizures. This change in seizure type can happen for a number of reasons, including missing a dose of medication, not getting enough sleep, or simply the way their disorder develops; for example, maybe they have always had a small chance of having a tonic–clonic seizure.

We don't know exactly why seizure patterns change over time. The current theory is that the brain changes (such as reorganization of connections or a change in the concentrations of certain chemicals) may be responsible. So if your child's seizures become more frequent or more severe, a neurologic checkup is advised. It may also be worthwhile to consider obtaining medication levels or a brain MRI.

3 | TYPES OF EPILEPSY: YOUR CHILD'S SYNDROME

When we talk about epilepsy, we aren't talking about one single disease or disorder, but an array of disorders in which seizures play a role. These disorders are referred to as *syndromes*. In diagnosing your child's particular epilepsy syndrome, the doctor will look at a number of factors, including the types of seizure or seizures your child has experienced, how old your child was when the seizures began, and the results of any electroencephalogram (EEG) results, if available. Knowing which epilepsy syndrome your child has is important for a number of reasons. First, the overall prognosis for your child can be better gauged. Second, your doctor may be able to tell about how long the seizures will persist. Finally, knowing the syndrome can give your child's doctors an indication of what medications or other treatments are likely to help. In this chapter, you'll find information on what defines a number of pediatric epilepsy syndromes. We've put febrile seizures first—since even when recurring, they're considered a seizure disorder rather than epilepsy—followed by a largely alphabetical listing of the types of epilepsy in children. In some of the descriptions, you'll see references to specific drugs. These drugs are discussed in detail in Chapter 10.

FEBRILE SEIZURES

Tommy was 14 months old. He caught a bad cold from a child in his playgroup, resulting in a fever and runny nose. He was taking a nap when his mother heard a strange banging sound. She ran into his room, and his whole body was stiff and shaking. It lasted less than five minutes, the longest five minutes of her life. He has never had another episode like this, and doesn't need any seizure medication. ■ ■ ■

Febrile seizures occur in 2 to 5 percent of children, some who come from families with a hereditary tendency toward these seizures. The peak age for the first febrile seizure is 18 months, but febrile seizures may start anytime between six months and six years. Typically, this kind of seizure occurs when a healthy child with normal development has a viral illness marked by high fever. As the child's temperature rapidly rises, he experiences a generalized tonic–clonic seizure. Most febrile seizures last less than five minutes. In most instances, hospitalization is not necessary, although a prompt medical consultation is essential after the first seizure to be sure that the seizure is not due to a brain infection or other cause. Chances of another seizure vary from 50 percent (if the seizure occurred before the child was one year old) to 25 percent (if the seizure occurred after that age). Other risk factors for recurrence refine the risk (see later in this chapter).

These seizures are not considered epilepsy, and the prognosis for children with febrile seizures is excellent. The vast majority will not have seizures without fever after age six, though a small number (only 2–3 percent) will go on to develop epilepsy. Risk factors for developing epilepsy after febrile seizures include abnormal development before the febrile seizure, complex febrile seizures (seizures lasting longer than 15 minutes, more than one seizure in 24 hours, or focal seizures), and a history of epilepsy in a parent or a sibling. If none of these risk factors are present, the child's chances of later developing epilepsy are similar to the chances of a child within the general population, or 0.5 to 1 percent. If one risk factor is present, the chances of later epilepsy are 5 percent; if two or more risk factors are present, the chances of later epilepsy are 5 to more than 10 percent.

Very rarely, febrile seizures that last more than 30 minutes may cause scar tissue in the temporal lobe and possibly chronic epilepsy. For this reason, parents of children with febrile seizures, especially those at high risk for recurrent febrile seizures or those who have had a prolonged febrile seizure, often keep "rescue" medication on hand. These medications, such as rectal diazepam or intranasal midazolam, can stop febrile seizures that last longer than a specified time (such as one to five minutes, depending on specific features of the patient's history). The decision to use rescue medications, and if so, how to use them, is complex and requires careful discussion with a doctor.

Studies show that febrile seizures cannot be prevented by baths, applying cool cloths to the child's head or body, or using fever-reducing medications such as acetaminophen (Tylenol) or ibuprofen (Advil, Motrin), despite the intuition of most parents and pediatricians. While acetaminophen and ibuprofen are safe and can help to reduce fever and discomfort, they do not prevent the seizures. Aspirin should not be given to young children.

Children who have had more than three febrile seizures or prolonged febrile seizures, or who have seizures when they have no fever, may benefit from daily medication. The role of benzodiazepine drugs such as diazepam or clonazepam at the time of fever and prevent recurrent febrile seizures is not well established. Most children with febrile seizures need no medication at all, and the seizures go away by age six.

COMMON EPILEPSY SYNDROMES

Benign Rolandic Epilepsy

Right after Timmy fell asleep, we heard a thud in his room. We rushed in and saw him on the floor having a whole-body seizure. The next day, the pediatrician asked if Timmy had ever had any tingling or jerking movements. We were shocked when Timmy said yes and explained that sometimes his tongue would tingle or his cheek would jerk. The doctor did an EEG and diagnosed Timmy with rolandic epilepsy, saying that Timmy didn't have to be treated. That's what we wanted to hear. He had one other milder seizure a few months later. It woke us up, but he couldn't talk because the side of his mouth was twitching and he was drooling. It's been five years now, and, except for a few tingles and twitches, Timmy has been doing great. ■ ■ ■

Benign rolandic epilepsy is a common childhood epilepsy syndrome, marked by seizures that usually begin between 2 and 10 years of age and a characteristic EEG pattern (Figure 3.1). A hereditary factor may contribute. The most characteristic type of benign rolandic epilepsy attack is a focal motor (twitching) or sensory (numbness or tingling sensation) seizure that involves one side of the face or tongue (the side can change from one seizure to the next) and may spread to the hand or cause garbled speech; in some cases, the attack is a tonic–clonic seizure instead. Seizures in benign rolandic epilepsy usually occur while a child is sleeping or is transitioning into or out of sleep. The seizures are often infrequent or occur in clusters of several per week followed by none for six months or longer.

Children with benign rolandic epilepsy have higher rates of attention deficit, reading comprehension, and language disorders than typical children. These problems are often transient and resolve as the child grows up.

Some patients benefit from medication—low to moderate doses of a drug that is often administered only after dinner or at bedtime—to keep the episodes under control. Patients needing medication tend to include children who also have daytime or recurrent tonic–clonic seizures, a learning or cognitive disorder, or multiple seizures at night that cause tiredness in the morning. The value of antiepileptic drugs (AEDs) for learning disorders has not been established. A big reason for AEDs is the child's fear of seizures—the choking feeling and inability to call for help may be terrifying. If a drug is needed, it can almost always be discontinued by age 15, at which point this type of epilepsy spontaneously resolves. The long-range outcome is excellent and children with rolandic epilepsy grow up to be normal adults who are seizure-free.

Childhood Absence Epilepsy

Childhood absence epilepsy is another common epilepsy syndrome, usually beginning between ages four and eight years in healthy children. One-third of childhood absence epilepsy patients come from families with a history of

FIGURE 3.1: An EEG reveals centrotemporal spikes (abnormal epilepsy waves recorded over the central and temporal regions) from a boy with benign rolandic epilepsy. The labels on the left side of the figure indicate the area of the brain from which each recording was obtained.

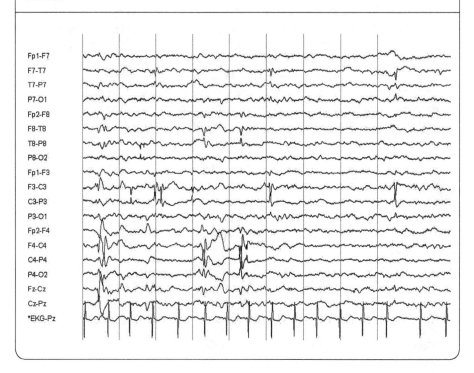

epilepsy. Children with this syndrome usually exhibit brief staring spells that begin and end suddenly and that tend to last between 3 and 20 seconds. The staring spells often cluster with repetitive seizures and can occur hundreds of times a day. Sometimes fluttering or jerking movements of the eyelids or eyebrows, or other automatic movements, accompany the spells. Children with childhood absence epilepsy tend to have higher rates of academic and social issues in later childhood than children in control groups.

An EEG is helpful in diagnosing and treating childhood absence epilepsy, since EEGs of children with the syndrome show a characteristic spike-and-wave pattern. The seizures and this pattern can usually be brought on by hyperventilation. In rare cases where the EEG shows polyspikes (two or more spikes before a slow wave), it can indicate that there is a lower chance of the child's seizures being controllable by medication and a lower chance of outgrowing epilepsy.

The most effective treatment for childhood absence epilepsy is medication (ethosuximide is the first choice, although lamotrigine and valproate are also effective). For most children with childhood absence epilepsy, the prognosis is very good: more than two-thirds will outgrow their epilepsy and fewer than 25 to 50 percent go on to have even one tonic–clonic seizure. Some patients later develop juvenile myoclonic epilepsy.

Juvenile Absence Epilepsy

Juvenile absence epilepsy most often begins when a child is between the ages of 10 and 16. Absence seizures are the principal seizure type in children with JAE, though both myoclonic and tonic–clonic seizures are involved more commonly than with childhood absence epilepsy. The EEG in these children often shows generalized spike-and-wave discharges. Unlike the single spike present in childhood absence epilepsy, a juvenile absence epilepsy EEG tends to show polyspikes, a marker for a more difficult-to-control and more likely convulsive epilepsy syndrome. Flashing lights will activate the EEG spikes or cause seizures (photosensitive epilepsy) in a third of children with JAE cases.

Juvenile absence epilepsy is treated with the same medications as childhood absence epilepsy, but since there is a greater chance that the child will develop myoclonic or tonic–clonic seizures, many doctors do not use ethosuximide as the first choice, as it is only effective for absence seizures. In 50 percent of juvenile absence epilepsy patients, the seizures eventually stop and the syndrome goes into remission.

Juvenile Myoclonic Epilepsy

Miranda has had these little jerks since she was 12, but she assumed everybody had them. They never really bothered her until one almost made her fall. She was put on medication for a few years, and then the drugs were stopped. During college, whenever she stayed up all night or drank too much, the next day she would get lots of the jerks, and sometimes a big seizure too. ■ ■ ■

Juvenile myoclonic epilepsy is a syndrome that usually begins around puberty, or less often in early adulthood. Although the syndrome may have a genetic basis, in most patients no first-degree relatives (parents, siblings, children) are affected. Girls are more commonly affected. Myoclonic seizures are the predominant seizure type, but are often very minor and not recognized. Most patients also have tonic–clonic seizures and some have a past or current history of absence seizures. The seizures happen most frequently in the early morning, soon after the child wakes up. They can be provoked by sudden awakening (say, by a loud phone) or if the child awakens and then rushes out of bed. A third of patients are photosensitive, with seizures triggered by flickering lights (such as the sun shining through trees). The seizures can also be provoked by factors such as reading, decision making, or calculations (see "Reflex Epilepsies" section). Patients with this syndrome sometimes display cognitive and behavioral problems that reflect mild dysfunction of frontal lobe "executive functions" such as planning and abstract reasoning, judgment, and inability to regulate reflexive or impulsive actions.

With this syndrome, the EEG shows a spike-and-wave pattern or polyspikes and waves pattern from both sides of the brain (generalized epilepsy waves).

In most children with juvenile myoclonic epilepsy, the seizures are easily controlled with drugs. Valproate is the treatment of choice but is not recommended for use during pregnancy; it can cause weight gain, hair loss, endocrine disorders, and other problems. Many patients are well controlled with other medications. Although this disorder is lifelong for most, at least 20 percent of juvenile myoclonic epilepsy patients outgrow epilepsy and can come off the medication and be seizure-free.

Frontal Lobe Epilepsy

Cassie's head starts jerking toward the right side. She tries to stop it but can't. Then her right hand goes up and her head turns toward the hand. She may stay in that position for half a minute and then it's over, or it may turn into a big seizure. ▪ ▪ ▪

Usually, Lucas doesn't get any warning, he just has tonic–clonic seizures. Occasionally he says there is a strange feeling in his head but it's only for a second before his seizure. ▪ ▪ ▪

I spend the night watching my daughter sleep sometimes. She'll have 5 or 10 seizures in a single night. The seizures are short, usually less than 20 seconds during which her body rocks as if she is adjusting her position in the bed, makes a strange throat sound, and then she may start to make kicking movements with her legs, as if she is riding a bicycle. She may not have any more seizures for a month or two. ▪ ▪ ▪

Craig has had the same giggling fits for more than a decade. Now they occur mainly when he is exercising or stressed. He makes a weird smirk and giggles for a few seconds. He can cover it up and people don't know. If he misses his medications, he might have a bigger seizure. ▪ ▪ ▪

Frontal lobe epilepsy is the second most common type of focal epilepsy, after temporal lobe epilepsy (discussed in the following "Temporal Lobe Epilepsy" section). The brain's large frontal lobes control a person's movement and also serve cognitive and behavioral functions. When a seizure affects the motor areas of the frontal lobes, the result is often jerking movements or stiffening—or occasionally weakness—on the opposite side of the body. When a seizure arises in the cognitive or behavioral areas, it can cause psychic effects (e.g., difficulty producing words or the emotion of fear), symptoms due to changes in the involuntary nervous system (e.g., related to sweating or heart rate), or other symptoms. In some cases, symptoms only occur when the seizure discharge spreads to other areas.

Seizures beginning in the frontal lobe usually last less than a minute and are followed by less confusion or tiredness than those from the temporal lobe. They can occur in a cluster or series, are much more likely to occur during sleep than temporal lobe seizures, and are more likely to include strange automatisms such as bicycling movements, screaming, or pelvic thrusting. If your child has a frontal lobe seizure, he may remain fully aware, even as his arms and legs move wildly. These focal seizures rarely cause laughing (*gelastic seizures*) or crying (*dacrystic seizures*). Laughing seizures may involve giggling, smirking, or fully developed laughter, with or without the emotion of joy. They can occur as simple or complex partial seizures and are seen in patients with frontal or temporal seizures or seizures arising from the hypothalamus (see Chapter 6). Because of their strange nature, frontal lobe seizures can be misdiagnosed as nonepileptic seizures.

It's possible to use clinical observations to diagnose frontal lobe seizures and to differentiate them from temporal lobe seizures, and recording one on video EEG can help with diagnosis. A magnetic resonance imaging (MRI) scan may provide evidence for where the seizure began and the cause. Causes include cortical malformations (e.g., cortical dysplasia) and brain injuries.

Frontal lobe seizures are treated with the medications prescribed for focal seizures, and may also be treated surgically or with vagus nerve stimulation or responsive neural stimulation (RNS) (see Chapter 14). Dietary therapies (see Chapter 11) are also sometimes used.

Reflex Epilepsies

It was only later that we realized that Joey was sitting under a flickering fluorescent light when he had his first seizure. All three of his seizures have happened in the presence of flashing or flickering lights. Once he had a seizure while in a car that was driving through a shaded area where the light flickered through leaves and branches. Now we give him dark blue sunglasses, and he keeps his head down in these kinds of settings, but he still has the seizures. ■ ■ ■

Reflex epilepsies are brought on by specific triggers—usually environmental. The most common form of reflex epilepsy is photosensitive epilepsy, a generalized epilepsy that often begins in childhood and is usually outgrown before adulthood. In photosensitive epilepsy, flashing lights can elicit absence, myoclonic, or tonic–clonic seizures. While people with photosensitive epilepsy are advised to avoid flashing lights, this is not always easy. Common experiences, such as riding a bike as sunshine flickers through the trees, can be provocative. For some people, certain rates of blinking or colors are most likely to provoke seizures. Video games and disco lights can also provoke these seizures, but this is rare (see Chapter 17); video and TV games or viewing and disco lights do not affect other epilepsies.

Other environmental triggers in reflex epilepsy include sounds such as a loud startling noise, certain types of music, or a person's voice; being touched, especially if it is unexpected; doing arithmetic; reading; and certain movements, such as writing. Internal triggers such as thinking about specific topics or experiencing a particular emotion can also provoke seizures, and mental excitement or stress can lower the seizure threshold for some patients with these syndromes. Most of the seizures involved in reflex epilepsy are generalized, although some are focal.

Because environmental triggers may be unavoidable or because nonreflex seizures also occur, many children with reflex epilepsy require treatment, often in the form of low doses of medications that include valproate, clonazepam, and carbamazepine. Some children, especially those with easily controlled seizures, outgrow this syndrome.

Temporal Lobe Epilepsy

I get the strangest feeling; most of it can't be put into words. At first, the whole world suddenly seems more real; it's as though everything becomes crystal clear. Then I feel as if I'm here but not here, kind of like being in a dream. It's as if I've lived through this moment many times before. I hear what people say, but they don't make sense. I know not to talk during the episode, since if I do I say foolish things. Sometimes I think I'm talking but later people tell me that I didn't say anything. The entire episode lasts a minute or two. ▪ ▪ ▪

Temporal lobe epilepsy is the most common focal epilepsy syndrome, and its seizures produce an incredibly wide spectrum of symptoms that can be hard even for articulate adults to describe. As a result, it's easy for parents to fail to recognize these symptoms in their children. Yet certain patterns link most patients with this syndrome, including sensations in the abdomen that rise to the chest or head. A person experiencing this kind of seizure will often sense a mixture of different emotions, thoughts, and experiences, some strangely familiar or oddly foreign. In some cases, a series of old memories resurfaces; in others, the person may feel as if everything—including his home and family—is strange. Hallucinations of voices, music, people, smells, or tastes may occur.

These sensations vary in intensity and quality but tend to be fairly consistent between seizures in the same individual. Some people experience these seizures in a form so mild that they barely notice, while others experience seizures that bring on clearly noticeable fright, intellectual fascination, or occasionally pleasure.

Fyodor Dostoyevsky, the Russian novelist, suffered from temporal lobe seizures and vividly described them in his novels. In this passage from one of his novels, a character named Prince Myshkin dwells on his seizure episodes:

He remembered that during his epileptic fits, or rather immediately preceding them, he had always experienced a moment or two when his whole heart, and mind, and body seemed to wake up with vigour and light; when he became filled with joy and hope, and all his anxieties seemed to be swept away for ever; these moments were but presentiments, as it were, of the one final second … in which the fit came upon him. That second, of course, was inexpressible.

Complex partial (or dyscognitive) seizures, typically lasting 30 to 120 seconds, are the most common seizure type in people with temporal lobe epilepsy. Three-quarters of children with temporal lobe epilepsy also have simple partial seizures (auras) and half have tonic–clonic seizures at some time. Some children will only have simple partial seizures.

Seizures in people with this syndrome usually begin in the deeper portions of the temporal lobe, in areas that control emotions and memory (see Figure AA.3C). As a result, some individuals will have short-term memory problems, especially if seizures have occurred for many years or if the person has had multiple or prolonged tonic–clonic seizures. The underlying cause of epilepsy and medications can also play an important role in memory disorders.

In most cases, these seizures can be well controlled with medication. If drugs are not effective, surgery can often control seizures. A specialized diet (the modified Atkins diet, discussed in Chapter 11), or responsive neurostimulation and vagus nerve stimulation (discussed in Chapter 14) may also be beneficial for some patients with temporal lobe epilepsy.

RARE EPILEPSY SYNDROMES

The following syndromes are uncommon and range in severity—some are quite mild and resolve easily, whereas others come with other serious symptoms and seizures are tougher to control. Some are associated with serious problems, such as intellectual disability, autism, and psychiatric disorders, which affect the child's life as much if not more than the seizures.

Benign Myoclonic Epilepsy of Infancy or Early Childhood

In this syndrome, children, predominantly boys between the ages of four months and three years, develop myoclonic seizures primarily affecting the head, eyes, and arms. Children with this syndrome don't typically get other types of seizures, although if the myoclonic seizures arise in clusters, they may impair consciousness.

The EEG shows generalized spike-and-wave discharges in these children. Antiepilepsy drugs such as valproate and clobazam are usually effective as treatments, and children virtually always outgrow this disorder.

Doose Syndrome (Myoclonic Astatic Epilepsy)

This generalized epilepsy disorder occurs in healthy children between six months and six years of age, often in families with a history of epilepsy. The predominant seizures are myoclonic, atonic drop attacks, and myoclonic–atonic (myoclonic astatic) seizures. The atonic (drop) seizures are key for diagnosis. A very common presentation is for a child to have many short myoclonic seizures followed by drop seizures. These children may also develop tonic–clonic, absence seizures, and tonic seizures. Prolonged seizures (known as status epilepticus) are common. Boys are twice as likely to have Doose syndrome as girls.

An EEG taken between a child's Doose seizures is often normal initially, but goes on to show generalized spike-and-wave discharges. Drugs used to treat generalized epilepsy are often effective with Doose patients. The ketogenic or modified Atkins diets tend to be useful as well. About half of the children with Doose syndrome outgrow it, but half have a persistent and often disabling disorder.

Generalized Epilepsy Febrile Seizures Plus

Generalized epilepsy febrile seizures plus (GEFS+), also called epilepsy febrile seizures plus (EFS+), is a syndrome with diverse clinical features caused by various genetic abnormalities (most commonly in the SCN1A gene). Many patients inherit this from a parent. Often more than one person in the family will be affected with some combination of febrile or afebrile seizures. Many doctors only diagnose GEFS+ in children with a family history. Again, the seizures vary from child to child: some have only simple febrile seizures that end before age six, whereas others have febrile seizures that are prolonged or recur up to age 11. Some families even have children with Dravet syndrome (see following section) as part of the spectrum. Other seizure types that people with GEFS+ may experience include absence, myoclonic, atonic, and focal seizures. Some patients' experiences with GEFS+ are very mild; others have seizures that are more difficult to control. Overall, about one-third have febrile seizures only, one-third have tonic–clonic seizures in adolescence, and one-third have other epilepsy types.

The EEG for a child with this syndrome may be normal or may show generalized epilepsy wave activity, usually most abundant in sleep; focal epilepsy waves may also be seen. Commercial labs can test for gene mutations that cause GEFS+. Mutations in the SCN1A gene can range widely in their effects—from causing only febrile seizures to GEFS+ to Dravet syndrome (see the following section).

Dravet Syndrome (Severe Myoclonic Epilepsy of Infancy/SMEI)

Dravet syndrome typically begins in the first year of a child's life with prolonged febrile seizures. (Sometimes routine vaccinations can cause fevers, and sometimes those fevers provoke seizures in those with Dravet syndrome. However, vaccines do *not* cause Dravet syndrome. Children with epilepsy, including those with Dravet syndrome, should be closely monitored after vaccinations rather than postponing or declining vaccinations.) Between ages one to two years, multiple seizure types emerge and are often treatment resistant. Initially, the seizures are generalized or unilateral clonic; later they will likely be myoclonic and partial (focal) seizures. Photosensitivity is common in early years and seizure frequency tends to diminish with age. Though this syndrome shares features with Lennox–Gastaut syndrome (see "Lennox–Gastaut Syndrome" section), fever-triggered seizures, an earlier age of onset (around six months of age) and infrequent occurrence of drop seizures help distinguish Dravet from this other disorder. Dravet also shares similarities with Doose syndrome, as children with Doose and Dravet both experience febrile convulsive seizures—but children with Doose syndrome usually have seizure onset after age one year, have frequent drop seizures, and do not show localized sharp waves on EEG and do not develop focal seizures. Intellectual disability, behavioral and sleep problems, and unsteady walking develop in most children with Dravet syndrome; autism occurs in approximately 25 percent. Seizures are often provoked by hot temperature, light (flashing or bright sun), and visual patterns.

Most children with Dravet's show abnormalities in their sodium channel genes (SCN1A, SCN1B, SCN2A) or other genes (GABRA1, STXBP1, PCDH19). These mutations are usually not present in either parent. Milder abnormalities in the SCN1A gene occur in patients with GEFS+ syndrome (see "Generalized Epilepsy Febrile Seizures Plus" section). The genetic abnormalities that cause most cases of Dravet can be detected in tests done by several commercial laboratories. An EEG can be helpful in Dravet, often showing features of both generalized and localized (partial) epilepsy waves at different times.

Treatment for Dravet syndrome is often challenging, and the disorder is lifelong. A number of antiepilepsy drugs as well as diet therapy can help, but no therapy is highly effective. AEDs that act primarily on sodium channels (such as lamotrigine, carbamazepine, phenytoin) often aggravate seizure activity in children with Dravet. Prolonged seizures and status epilepticus are common, often requiring rescue medications, which may be given close to seizure onset, rather than after three to five minutes, if the child's seizures are almost always prolonged. Finally, there's a growing interest in the role of cannabidiol (CBD) and other mixed cannabis (marijuana) products—predominantly CBD and tetrahydrocannibinol (THC)—as treatments for children with Dravet syndrome and other refractory epilepsies.

Electrical Status Epilepticus of Slow Wave Sleep or Continuous Spike and Wave in Slow Wave Sleep

Electrical status epilepticus of slow wave sleep (ESES) and continuous spike and wave in slow wave sleep (CSWS) share some EEG and clinical features, and the names are used inconsistently. We will consider them interchangeable. Both syndromes are rare and often associated with a regression of language, memory, and other cognitive and behavioral skills. Onset is typically between ages five and seven, and these syndromes are slightly more common in boys. Some children diagnosed with these disorders have shown severe developmental delays since early life, and the EEG findings are identified long after the developmental problems. In these instances, it is hard to know if the symptoms shown on the EEG contributed to or caused the developmental delays or if an underlying brain disorder caused both the delays and EEG findings. At the other end of the spectrum are children with benign rolandic epilepsy whose EEG in sleep shows extremely frequent epilepsy activity, and thus may meet the criteria for ESES. These children may be neurologically normal or have only mild learning, attention deficit, or other disorders.

The key diagnostic tool, as mentioned previously, is the EEG, which usually shows nearly continuous generalized epilepsy waves (slow spike-and-wave discharges) or, less often, localized epilepsy waves in nonrapid eye movement sleep (non-REM; the phase of sleep when few dreams occur). One-third of children with these syndromes have MRIs that show abnormalities such as decreased brain size (atrophy) or malformations of cortical development.

The prognosis for seizure control is usually very good, but the challenge is clearing up the EEG spikes in sleep. Some patients respond well to steroids, as with Landau–Kleffner syndrome (see "Landau–Kleffner Syndrome" section). Some respond to high doses of benzodiazepines given over short periods.

Landau–Kleffner Syndrome

Landau–Kleffner syndrome causes acquired aphasia (the loss of previously acquired language abilities) and affects boys more often than girls. Typically with this syndrome, a child between ages three and eight gradually experiences language problems, with or without seizures. The problems usually involve auditory comprehension (understanding spoken language), but speaking ability can also be affected. This syndrome's related simple partial motor and tonic–clonic seizures are infrequent, often nocturnal, and easily controlled with medications.

The boundaries that define Landau–Kleffner syndrome are imprecise. One variant, for example, involves children whose language function is delayed or never develops. In this version, the epilepsy waves likely contribute to or cause the language disorder before language ability has begun to develop.

The epilepsy waves in children with Landau–Kleffner syndrome are sometimes localized over language areas but may be more generalized, and in both cases they are activated by sleep. As a result, taking an EEG during sleep is the key to diagnosis. A normal EEG that has been taken when the child is awake will not rule out this disorder.

Antiepilepsy drugs are ineffective in treating the language disorder. Steroids, however, may improve the EEG abnormalities and also the language problems. A type of epilepsy surgery, multiple subpial transections (see Chapter 14), can be helpful in select cases.

Infantile Spasms

At first we thought Chris was just having the little body jerks when he was moved or startled, like our other children had when they were infants. But then the jerks became more violent, and his tiny body spasmed forward and his arms flew apart—and we knew something was wrong. These episodes only lasted a few seconds each, but they started to occur in groups lasting a few minutes. It was so hard to see our young baby going through this. ■ ■ ■

Infantile spasms (also known as West Syndrome) is a form of epilepsy that begins between 3 and 12 months of age and usually resolves by the age of two to four years. Each of these seizures, or spasms, consists of a sudden jerk followed by stiffening. During some spells known as *jackknife seizures,* the child's arms are flung out as his body bends forward. Other spells are more subtle, with movements limited to the child's neck or other particular body parts. Sixty percent of the infants with infantile spasms have suffered a brain disorder or injury—such as birth trauma that resulted in oxygen deprivation or a genetic disorder such as tuberous sclerosis. The other 40 percent have had normal development and brain structure when spasms begin. Genetic disorders likely contribute to some of the "unknown" cases.

The prognosis for seizure control and development in cases of infantile spasms depends on the underlying cause of the seizures, the child's intellectual and neurological development before the seizures began, and whether the seizures come under control quickly. Overall, the sooner a child begins therapy for infantile spasms and the sooner the seizures and the abnormal EEG patterns are controlled, the better the outcome.

Treatment might include hormonal, drug, and dietary therapies. Injections of the adrenocorticotropic hormone (ACTH) stop seizures in more than half of children with infantile spasms. Side effects depend on the dose used (the dose diminishes as the therapy progresses), the duration of therapy, and the baby's sensitivity, and can range from mild to serious. For most children, the benefits of ACTH outweigh the side effects, but the side effects should be monitored closely. Vigabatrin (Sabril) is often used as the initial therapy as well, because it is safe for short-term use and effective in many. Prednisone is another therapy with effects similar to those of ACTH. It is an oral therapy that does not require injections; however, some studies suggest that it is not as effective as ACTH.

Infantile spasms will stop in more than 90 percent of children by the age of five years. However, other seizure types often develop later on. One-fifth of patients with infantile spasms, for example, go on to develop Lennox–Gastaut syndrome.

Lennox–Gastaut Syndrome

When the doctors told me Tommy's diagnosis was Lennox–Gastaut syndrome, the words had no meaning to me. So I went to the Internet and ended up in tears. The prognosis sounded totally hopeless; there was no future. Ten years later, though, Tommy's seizures are under much better control. He loves his special ed classes, has lots of friends, is an incredibly important part of our family, and gives us all great pleasure. ▪ ▪ ▪

As the parents of a child with Lennox–Gastaut syndrome, we need lots of patience. Kathy has been on every medication, many of them three or four times. Nothing has controlled the seizures well. As the doctors upped the doses, she would undergo terrible personality changes, turn into a zombie, or look drunk. We finally came to accept the seizures and her mental handicaps. We now have part-time help at home so that we and our other kids can lead a more normal life. As we let go of some our unrealistic hopes and accepted Kathy for who she is, our disappointment changed to joy. ▪ ▪ ▪

Lennox–Gastaut syndrome (LGS) is a severe form of epilepsy that usually first appears when a child is between one and six years of age, but it can begin later. It is defined by three features: difficult-to-control seizures, intellectual disability, and a slow spike-and-wave pattern on the EEG. The seizures involved are usually a combination of tonic, atypical absence, myoclonic, and tonic–clonic that can result in falls and injuries. Most children with the syndrome have mild to severe intellectual impairment and behavioral problems that can be attributed to a combination of the primary neurological disorder (e.g. genetic disorder or infection), seizures, and the drugs used to treat the syndrome.

Although seizures associated with LGS tend to be resistant to medication, these seizures vary greatly from child to child. Some children are able to achieve good, although rarely complete, seizure control with the help of a wide range of the drugs prescribed for both generalized and focal epilepsies. Others continue to have drop attacks, atypical absence, partial, and tonic–clonic seizures. Frequent seizures, especially those that cause falls, can lead to head injuries and the need for high doses of several of the drugs. Overall, for patients with poorly controlled seizures, it is best to avoid high doses of multiple antiepilepsy drugs, because they can intensify the behavioral, social, and intellectual problems. Many families prefer to tolerate slightly more frequent seizures and having a more alert, attentive child with a higher quality of life.

Vagus nerve stimulation or corpus callosotomy (see Chapter 14) is able to help some children with LGS. The ketogenic or modified Atkins diets are often effective in treating seizures in patients with LGS.

LGS usually persists into adulthood, and affected people often need to live in a residential group home when they want more independence or when their parents are no longer able to care for them. As children age, the characteristic features change: the EEG often changes to show multifocal spikes, and the main seizures become focal or tonic–clonic.

Ohtahara Syndrome

Ohtahara syndrome is a very rare, treatment-resistant epilepsy that begins in the first three months of a child's life, often in the first two weeks. It typically involves tonic seizures, but also can have spasms, focal, and myoclonic seizures. Children with this syndrome have severe cognitive, motor, and other developmental delays.

The EEG signature of this syndrome—a high-amplitude spike-and-wave burst followed by relative electrical silence—is critical in making the diagnosis. Abnormalities in several genes (STXBP1, CDKL5, and ARX, among more than 18 genes) can cause Ohtahara syndrome.

Common treatments include drugs, steroids, and dietary therapies. Even with these treatments, seizures often persist.

PCDH19

PCDH19 is a genetic disorder resulting from a mutation in the PCDH19 gene on the X chromosome. All affected individuals are girls. When males have the abnormal gene, they are largely unaffected, but can pass on the disorder to their daughters. Women with the abnormal gene have a 50 percent chance of passing it to their daughters and 50 percent chance of passing the gene to their sons. Seizures usually begin between ages three months to three years (average nine months). Affected girls have multiple seizure types, including tonic–clonic, tonic, atonic, myoclonic, and focal. Like Dravet syndrome, with which PCHD19 may be confused, seizures are often provoked by fever, can occur in clusters, and are difficult to control.

Progressive Myoclonic Epilepsies

After a few tonic–clonics, we started Avi on medication. Each drug worked for a while and then it stopped working. The jerks that we barely noticed before became more and more frequent. We tried more and more drugs, two or three at a time, and the number of seizures actually increased. The worst part was that Avi was slipping—he was changing. He was not as sharp and quick as he had been, and we blamed the drugs. It kept getting worse, including the onset of little seizures that caused his speech to sputter and hesitate, and his mind to turn on and off, as if someone was taking a light switch and flicking it up and down. ▪ ▪ ▪

Progressive myoclonic epilepsies are rare and involve myoclonic and tonic–clonic seizures that are difficult to control and associated with deteriorating neurologic function. The seizures may be triggered by movement or sensory stimuli (sound, touch, or visual). These epilepsies are usually caused by a variety of hereditary metabolic disorders, each of which have their own names (such as Lafora disease or Unvericht-Lundberg—you can see why the name progressive myoclonic epilepsy is used), but in some cases, their origins remain unknown. Genetic testing can often identify the abnormal gene.

Drugs for myoclonic and generalized tonic–clonic seizures, such as valproate, levetiracetam, zonisamide, and clobazam, can be useful in children with this disorder. Drug treatment is of limited benefit, however, because as the disorder progresses, the drugs become less effective and their side effects may become more severe. There are many different causes and the course and prognosis depend on the cause.

Rasmussen's Syndrome

Rasmussen's is a severe disorder that usually begins when a child is between 14 months and 14 years of age. It's defined by slowly progressive neurologic deterioration and simple partial and tonic–clonic seizures, which are often the first sign of the syndrome. Epilepsia partialis continua—a prolonged, almost continuous seizure with jerking of one side or just one muscle group—is also common in patients with Rasmussen's and responds poorly to medication.

Although Rasmussen's syndrome is rarely fatal, its effects are serious. One to three years after the seizures start, weakness and other neurologic problems often begin. Mild weakness of an arm or leg is the most common initial symptom after the seizures, but progressive weakness on one side (hemiparesis) and mental retardation are common. Aphasia can occur if the brain's language hemisphere is affected.

Serial computed tomography (CT) and MRI scans show a slow loss of brain substance in people with Rasmussen's. Though no definitive cause of the syndrome is known, it is probably an autoimmune disorder (a disorder in which antibodies are produced that battle against the body's own tissues) and may be triggered by a viral infection.

Though treatment with antiepilepsy drugs has disappointing results in these children, steroids and other immune-modulating therapies such as gamma globulin plasmapheresis sometimes help. In children with severe loss of function in the involved hemisphere, a surgical procedure called a functional hemispherectomy (see Chapter 14) can be successful. Most experts recommend hemispherectomy early in the course to prevent progression and involvement of the other hemisphere.

SELECTED DISORDERS IN WHICH EPILEPSY IS A MAJOR FEATURE

The following syndromes are uncommon or rare. Most are associated with high rates of intellectual disability, autism, and psychiatric disorders.

Aicardi Syndrome

Aicardi syndrome is a rare genetic syndrome affecting almost exclusively girls in which the large fiber bundle that connects two brain hemispheres, the corpus callosum, is partially or completely absent. These girls often have eye abnormalities. Epilepsy occurs in more than half of cases, often appearing as infantile spasms at first but then progressing into other seizure types. The seizures often persist despite antiepilepsy drug therapy. Both motor and cognitive developments are typically very impaired.

CDKL5

CDKL5 is a rare syndrome characterized by infantile spasms starting in the first six months of a child's life. The syndrome is an atypical form of Rett syndrome (see "Rett Syndrome" section) caused by a mutation in the CDKL5 gene. Older children with the disorder tend to have tonic–clonic seizures lasting several minutes, during which the stiffening of the tonic phase coincides with superimposed "tremor/vibratory" movements, followed by a clonic phase that ends with myoclonic jerks in the hands and feet.

The EEG for children with CDKL5 usually shows generalized epilepsy waves. The seizures associated with CDKL5 tend to be resistant to treatment.

Dup15q Syndrome

In this syndrome, a duplication of part of chromosome 15 (known as q11.2-13.1) causes motor and cognitive developmental delays that include autism, behavioral disorders, and epilepsy. A child with Dup15q often has a button nose, deep-set eyes, and eye folds. Early in life, the child will have hypotonia (poor muscle tone), which is often replaced by spasticity (increased tone) in later life.

This syndrome often includes several types of seizures that are frequently difficult to control. These include myoclonic, tonic, and tonic–clonic seizures.

FOXG1 Syndrome

Like, CDKL5, FOXG1 syndrome is a variation of Rett syndrome (see "Rett Syndrome" section) and due to mutations in the gene FOXG1. Children with FOXG1 exhibit severe developmental delays, lack of speech, deficient growth, small head size, stereotypic movements, and epilepsy. The seizures—tonic–clonic and/or complex partial—often begin between ages three months and six years.

The EEG for these children can show generalized or focal epilepsy activity. An MRI may also show abnormalities. Those with duplications of FOXG1 often develop infantile spasms, respond to ACTH therapy, and do not require long-term antiepileptic drug therapy. Those with deletions or mutations in the FOXG1 gene usually require long-term antiepilepsy drugs.

Hypothalamic Hamartoma

Hypothalamic hamartomas are small benign tumors in the base of the brain that affect the hypothalamus (see Figure AA.1C) and cause partial seizures (with laughing as a frequent feature); in many cases, there is early puberty, irritability, aggression, and intellectual disability. Simple and complex partial seizures and also secondary generalized tonic–clonic seizures can occur. Children with this disorder are often short in stature and have mild abnormalities in their physical features (dysmorphisms).

An MRI is necessary for diagnosing hypothalamic hamartoma.

Surgery (removal or laser ablation) or gamma knife radiosurgery can reduce or control seizures in many cases. Antiepilepsy medication can also be beneficial, but is often insufficient to fully control seizures. Drugs aimed at hormonal and behavioral problems may be helpful.

Mitochondrial Disorders

Mitochondria are the energy factories of a cell. Abnormalities in the function of these factories cause metabolic disorders that affect different parts of the body, including muscles and the brain. Several of these mitochondrial disorders result in myoclonic, absence, and tonic–clonic seizures, as well as other neurologic problems such as stroke-like episodes, hearing loss, dementia, headaches, vomiting, unsteadiness, and problems with exercise.

Mitochondrial disorders are diagnosed by testing a child's blood and spinal fluid. Commercial tests can test for specific genetic disorders from a blood sample and are becoming more sensitive. In addition to antiepilepsy drugs, children with mitochondrial disorders often benefit from "mito cocktails" that include supplements such as coenzyme Q10, L-carnitine, and B vitamins.

Rett Syndrome

Rett is a syndrome that appears in early childhood and causes delays and regression of language, cognitive, and motor abilities. Because the gene defect is on the X chromosome, the vast majority of Rett patients are girls, and these girls tend to display distinctive physical features: small head size (microcephaly), small hands and feet, and repetitive hand movements. Most children have normal development in the first year of life and then regress, showing features of autism after age one. Seizures—predominately complex partial and tonic–clonic—occur in more than half of Rett patients, usually beginning between ages 3 and 16.

More than 90 percent of people with Rett have a mutation on their MECP2 gene. Duplication of the MECP2 gene can also cause epilepsy, as well as severe cognitive and motor delays (beginning in infancy), spasticity, and abnormal movements.

Ring 20 (r20) Syndrome

Ring 20 is a rare chromosomal anomaly that happens when there are two breaks on chromosome 20 resulting in a circular chromosome. The syndrome can appear in a child at birth or later. Patients with this syndrome often develop treatment-resistant absence seizures that are often prolonged, as well as focal seizures. Cognitive and behavioral disorders are very frequent.

The seizures associated with Ring 20 are often difficult to control, though in some cases antiepileptic drugs help (such as valproic acid and lamotrigine in combination). A characteristic seizure type is a prolonged spike wave event with decreased but still present consciousness.

Tuberous Sclerosis Complex

Tuberous sclerosis complex (TSC) is a genetic disorder usually caused by mutations in the TSC1 or TSC2 genes involving a cell growth pathway. Most cases result from mutations that are acquired when DNA is copied in the parents' sperm or egg or after conception, although some are inherited. This disorder results in abnormal tissue development and benign tumors in multiple organs, including the brain. Seizures occur in nearly 90 percent of cases. Many young children experience infantile spasms that respond to the drug vigabatrin. Older children often show mixed focal and generalized seizures, including simple and complex partial, tonic and atonic, and tonic–clonic.

Treatments for TSC include standard therapies for the specific seizure types, including dietary therapies. Surgical therapy can be very effective in cases where a single seizure focus is identified and also when seizures are coming from multiple sites, albeit with a primary goal of reducing rather than fully controlling episodes.

Once your child's particular syndrome is diagnosed, your family's path toward dealing with the epilepsy can begin, since knowing the syndrome will help you and your medical team narrow down the treatment options. Pinning down what caused the epilepsy—something that's not always possible—can also help in determining treatment. We'll look at the causes of epilepsy in Chapter 4.

4 | CAUSES OF EPILEPSY

As a parent, it's natural to want to know the cause of your child's epilepsy. Knowing this cause can provide some comfort—simply in the fact that it's a firm bit of knowledge about your child's condition—but more important, it can help doctors determine a treatment plan. Unfortunately, there isn't always an easily discernable reason that a particular child has epilepsy. This is largely because the causes can be so varied—technically, anything that injures a person's brain or disrupts the brain's electrical or chemical balance can potentially cause epilepsy. The current thinking divides these varied causes into three broad categories: genetic, structural/metabolic (formerly called symptomatic), and unknown. This classification system can be reassuring to parents and doctors looking for easily digested answers, but it tends to oversimplify things, as a single case of epilepsy can fall into two or even all three categories. For example, a child's family history of epilepsy (genetic cause) increases her risk of developing epilepsy after a head injury (structural cause). Tuberous sclerosis is a genetic cause of epilepsy associated with structural brain abnormalities (tubers) and metabolic dysfunction in the brain's mTOR metabolic pathway in nerve cells, making it a genetic disorder with structural/metabolic features. Finally, unknown factors almost always influence the way a particular case of epilepsy is expressed and how it responds to treatment, even if the case's genetic or structural cause is well defined. In some instances, a patient's history, exam, and imaging are normal, but several family members have epilepsy and a genetic cause is strongly suspected but not confirmed. In many cases, we simply don't know.

Be aware that the cause of your child's epilepsy may be incorrectly identified, at least at first. This is very common, for a number of reasons. For example, many children have a history of a difficult birth delivery or have their first seizure shortly after a vaccination. A doctor or parents may see these factors as clues: the initial seizures in children with Dravet syndrome often begin after a vaccination, and many children and adults have their first seizures within weeks or months of a mild head injury (defined as a loss of consciousness for less than 10 minutes). But these factors can sometimes lead parents and doctors in the wrong direction. This is because although it's easy to assume a causal relationship between the vaccinations or a tough delivery or a minor head injury and the epilepsy, extensive studies show that vaccines, difficult deliveries, and mild head injuries do *not* cause epilepsy. So, while it's natural to feel a strong desire to identify a cause, it's also important to keep in mind that although this can lead to the right answer, it can also lead you down the wrong path.

THE THREE CATEGORIES OF CAUSES

Structural or metabolic causes: Epilepsies with structural causes stem from abnormalities in the brain's formation that can usually be seen on a neuroimaging test (an MRI or computed tomography, known as CT). These abnormalities can be the result of severe head injuries, scar tissue, problems of brain development, strokes, meningitis, and more. The cause is typically documented in the patient's clinical history (for example, head trauma with depressed skull fracture or prolonged loss of consciousness) and then also revealed on a neuroimaging test.

Metabolic causes of epilepsy involve disorders in the brain's or body's metabolic system (*metabolism* is the word for the chemical reactions that go on in all people's cells). These causes of epilepsy should be distinguished from metabolic causes of seizures, since any abnormalities in blood sugar (severe hypoglycemia or hyperglycemia), magnesium levels, or sodium (hyponatremia) levels can lead to seizures. Seizures that result from these abnormal levels are considered *provoked* seizures, and even if recurrent are not diagnosed as epilepsy. By contrast, metabolic causes of epilepsy feature "inborn errors of metabolism" (Tables 4.1 and 4.2). All types of

TABLE 4.1: METABOLIC CAUSES OF EPILEPSY

Category of Metabolic Disorder	Specific Forms
Energy deficiency	GLUT-1 deficiency, mitochondrial respiratory chain deficiency, carnitine deficiency
Vitamin or cofactor dependency	Biotinidase deficiency, pyridoxine-dependent, and pyridoxal phosphate–dependent epilepsy, folinic acid-responsive seizures, Menkes disease
Storage diseases	Tay-Sachs, GM1 gangliosidosis, Gaucher types 2 and 3, Sandhoff
Neurotransmitter disorders	GABA transaminase deficiency, nonketotic hyperglycinemia, succinic semialdehyde dehydrogenase deficiency

Note: *These are inborn errors of metabolism, typically resulting from genetic causes that can result in a variety of disorders affecting the body and brain, and in many cases, cause epilepsy.*

GABA, gamma-amino butyric acid; GLUT-1, glucose transporter protein 1.

focal and secondary generalized seizures, and even some generalized seizures such as tonic or myoclonic seizures, can result from either structural or metabolic causes.

Genetic causes: Thanks to advances in genetic testing, genetic abnormalities are emerging as a common cause of epilepsy. More than 90 "epilepsy genes" have been identified, and there are likely hundreds of other genes that influence a person's susceptibility to developing seizures and epilepsy. Genetic abnormalities can be inherited or arise as new mutations. New mutations are not present in either parent, while inherited disorders are most commonly from one parent (dominant mutations) or both parents (recessive mutations; each parent is a carrier). Rarely, an unaffected parent is a mosaic, meaning that the mutation is

TABLE 4.2: GENETIC CAUSES OF EPILEPSY

Seizure/Epilepsy Type	Genetic Disorder	Metabolic Disorder
Infantile spasms	Tuberous sclerosis	Biotinidase deficiency, Menkes' disease, mitochondrial disorders, organic acidurias, aminoacidopathies
Epilepsy with learning or behavioral disorder	ADSL, ALDH7A1, ARX, ATP1A2, ATP6AP2, CACNB4, CDKL5, CHRNA2, CHRNA4, CHRNA7, CHRNB2, CLN3, CLN5, CLN6, CLN8, CNTNAP2, CSTB, CTSD, DNAJC5, EFHC1, EPM2A, FOLR1, FOXG1, GABRA1, GABRG2, GAMT, GATM, GOSR2, GRIN2A, GRIN2B, KANSL1, KCNJ10, KCNQ2, KCNQ3, KCTD7, LGI1, LIAS, MAGI2, MBD5, MECP2, MEF2C, MFSD8, NHLRC1, NRXN1, PCDH19, PNKP, PNPO, POLG, PPT1, PRICKLE1, PRRT2, SCARB2, SCN1A, SCN1B, SCN2A, SCN8A, SLC25A22, SLC2A1, SLC9A6, SPTAN1, SRPX2, STXBP1, SYN1, TBC1D24, TCF4, TPP1 (CLN2), TSC1 & TSC2 (tuberous sclerosis), UBE3A, ZEB2	
Myoclonic-astatic seizures	SCN1A, SLC2A1	GLUT1-deficiency, NCL2

(continued)

TABLE 4.2: GENETIC CAUSES OF EPILEPSY (*CONTINUED*)

Seizure/Epilepsy Type	Genetic Disorder	Metabolic Disorder
Myoclonic seizures	ADSL, ALDH7A1, ARX, ATP1A2, ATP6AP2, CACNB4, CDKL5, CHRNA2, CHRNA4, CHRNA7, CHRNB2, CLN3, CLN5, CLN6, CLN8, CNTNAP2, CSTB, CTSD, DNAJC5, EFHC1, EPM2A, FOLR1, FOXG1, GABRA1, GABRG2, GAMT, GATM, GOSR2, GRIN2A, GRIN2B, KANSL1, KCNJ10, KCNQ2, KCNQ3, KCTD7, LGI1, LIAS, MAGI2, MBD5, MECP2, MEF2C, MFSD8, NHLRC1, NRXN1, PCDH19, PNKP, PNPO, POLG, PPT1, PRICKLE1, PRRT2, SCARB2, SCN1A, SCN1B, SCN2A, SCN8A, SLC25A22, SLC2A1, SLC9A6, SPTAN1, SRPX2, STXBP1, SYN1, TBC1D24, TCF4, TPP1 (CLN2), TSC1, TSC2, UBE3A, ZEB2	Nonketotic hyperglycinemia, mitochondrial disorders, GLUT1-deficiency, storage disorders
Progressive myoclonic epilepsies	CLN3, CLN5, CLN6, CLN8, CSTB, CTSD, DNAJC5, EPM2A, FOLR1, GOSR2, KCTD7, MFSD8, NHLRC1, PPT1, PRICKLE1, SCARB2, TPP1 (CLN2)	Lafora disease, MERRF, MELAS, Unverricht–Lundborg disease, sialidosis
Epilepsy with multi-focal seizures	SCN1A	NCL3, GLUT1-deficiency
Epilepsia partialis continua		Alpers disease, other mitochondrial disorders
Rett, Angelman, CDKL5	CDKL5, CNTAP2, FOXG1, MBD5, MECP2, MEF2C, NRXN1, SLC9A6, TCF4, UBE3A, ZEB2	

GLUT-1, glucose transporter protein 1.

found in only a portion of his or her cells, but they can transmit the mutation to a child who is affected.

Cytogenetic testing, which is used to identify chromosomal abnormalities such as trisomy 21 (Down syndrome) and Fragile X syndrome, can detect large duplications or deletions in chromosomes that can cause epilepsy. Chromosomal microarray testing is able to identify the small duplications or deletions in DNA that are referred to as *copy number variants*. Copy number variants are identified in up to 10 to 15 percent of patients with intellectual and developmental disabilities, many of whom have epilepsy. Other genetic tests include gene panels for specific types of seizures or epilepsies (infantile spasms, childhood-onset epilepsy, myoclonic epilepsy, progressive myoclonic epilepsy). People interested in having genetic tests done for epilepsy can have epilepsy gene panels performed by GeneDx (genedx.com), Ambry Genetics (ambrygen.com), or other companies. Whole exome sequencing can also be done; this process examines the DNA sequence of a person's approximately 20,000 protein-coding genes. One challenge of whole exome sequencing is that variants are frequently discovered that are not present in the general population, but their relationship to the child's epilepsy or other disorders is often uncertain. When such variants are found on chromosomal microarray, gene panels, and whole exome sequencing, the child's parents can be tested to confirm if the mutations are new (de novo) and thus not inherited from a parent, making them more likely to be causative than mutations inherited from a neurologically normal parent. A geneticist or genetic counselor is often critical to decipher the meaning of these test results.

Unknown causes: Epilepsies without known cause have also been referred to as idiopathic epilepsies, although this term is no longer recommended; it's best to simply say the cause is not known. Cases in which the cause is unknown include both generalized and focal epilepsies. We believe that unidentified genetic factors lower the seizure threshold in many of these patients. Epilepsy patients in whom the cause is unknown usually have no other disabilities.

CAUSES OF FOCAL (PARTIAL) VERSUS GENERALIZED EPILEPSIES

Knowing whether your child's seizures are focal or generalized can help you find the seizures' cause. If your child has a form of focal epilepsy, it probably is caused by a known or suspected disorder (a structural or metabolic cause) affecting one or more localized brain areas. If you child has generalized epilepsy, it may be the result of identified or suspected genetic factors (either inherited or new), even if no one else in the family has epilepsy. Many of the genes that cause epilepsy control cellular structures such as the body's ion channels and neurotransmitter receptors (see the following "Channelopathies" section). Again, the dividing line isn't firm. For example, hereditary factors and ion channel dysfunction can cause focal as well as generalized epilepsies. And generalized epilepsies may be "activated" by structural causes such as head injury.

Channelopathies: A Model of Generalized Epilepsy?

Ion channels are complex proteins that regulate the flow of charged atoms such as sodium or potassium across cell membranes. These channels are essential in keeping the balance of excitability in all cells, including nerve cells. Genetic changes in the structure of these channels—even the substitution of a single amino acid for another at a critical site—can disrupt the fine balance of nerve cell excitability and result in recurrent seizures. These disorders of ion channels, or *channelopathies*, are the most commonly recognized genetic cause of generalized epilepsy. Mutations in the sodium channel gene, SCN1A, can cause a spectrum of disorders, from febrile seizures to generalized epilepsy febrile seizures-plus (GEFS+) to Dravet syndrome (see Chapter 3).

Some ion channel disorders occur in large families where many members have epilepsy. The electroencephalograms (EEGs) of those patients show the classic generalized 3 to 5 Hz/sec spike-and-wave discharges (see Figure 5.3). However, most patients with generalized epilepsy do not have close relatives with epilepsy. The fact that these patients show similar EEG findings suggests that they may also have ion channel abnormalities.

Kindling: A Model of Focal Epilepsy

Patients often ask why an interval of years can pass between a brain injury or an abnormality of brain development and the first seizure. There is no single or simple answer to how epilepsy develops (the process of *epileptogenesis*). Indeed, there are undoubtedly many roads that lead to epilepsy. One experimental model, kindling, provides insights into one possible road and may answer the question of why those years-long intervals exist.

If an area of a mouse's or monkey's brain is stimulated once a day with a small electrical current, initially there may be no changes. After a week, there may be a small, local storm of electrical activity after the stimulation. After several weeks, the storm may spread to neighboring areas and the animal may show symptoms such as facial grimacing or blank staring. As the stimulation is repeated, the electrical storms and seizure symptoms become more intense, eventually causing a tonic–clonic seizure. Finally, in some animals, spontaneous seizures occur—that is, without the electrical stimulation. Thus, a "fire" has been "kindled" in the animal's brain. The similarity between the patterns of seizures, the EEG activity, and the changes found in the brains of kindled animals and in patients with focal epilepsy suggests that kindling may occur in humans. Thus, a brain injury triggers abnormal electrical currents, which may progress over months or years to cause seizures.

Causes of Focal Epilepsy

As mentioned earlier, generalized epilepsy is largely caused by genetic factors. Focal epilepsy is often caused by structural factors, and scientific studies of populations (epidemiologic studies) have identified many of these factors.

Table 4.3 lists the major risk factors. It is likely that genetic factors contribute to susceptibility to focal epilepsy and in some cases, can cause focal epilepsy.

Many other disorders that affect the brain, either primarily or as part of a more widespread problem, can cause epilepsy. These include autism, metabolic disorders (such as mitochondrial, amino acid, and storage disorders), chromosomal disorders (such as trisomy 21/Down syndrome, Fragile X, ring chromosome 20), and neurocutaneous disorders with neurologic and skin involvement (such as tuberous sclerosis, neurofibromatosis, and hypomelanosis of Ito).

TABLE 4.3: CAUSES OF EPILEPSY

Factors Associated with a 10-Fold or Greater Risk of Epilepsy

Infants with seizures in the first month of life

Head injury that causes one or more of the following:
  Loss of consciousness > 30 minutes
  Significant memory impairment after the injury
  Abnormalities such as weakness or impaired coordination
  Skull fracture

Infections
  Meningitis
  Encephalitis
  Cerebral abscess

Brain tumors

Cerebral palsy

Intellectual disability

Alzheimer's disease

Febrile status epilepticus

Stroke

Blood vessel malformations in the brain
  Arteriovenous malformations
  Cavernous angiomas

Alcohol abuse

Factors Associated with a 2–10-Fold or Greater Risk of Epilepsy

Use of illegal drugs such as heroin or cocaine

Family history of epilepsy or febrile seizures

Multiple sclerosis

Seizures occurring within days after head injury ("early posttraumatic seizures")

Epidemiologic studies show that there is no relationship between vaccination and epilepsy. In some cases, however, vaccination causes a fever that can provoke a febrile convulsion. This is common in patients with Dravet syndrome who may have a prolonged seizure after vaccination. We strongly recommend that children with epilepsy receive vaccinations. They can be monitored for fever and treated with acetaminophen or ibuprofen. Disorders such as measles or pertussis (whooping cough) can be severe or even deadly. Mild head injury, such as a concussion where consciousness is lost for less than 10 to 15 minutes, is not a cause of epilepsy.

Autoimmune disorders can cause epilepsy. These can affect the body, such as lupus erythematosus, antiphospholipid syndrome, rheumatic arthritis, and Sjögren's syndrome. Autoimmune encephalitis is a disorder of the immune system that can selectively affect the brain and cause seizures as well as other problems affecting speech, involuntary movements, and behavior. Specific antibodies that occur in this disorder are directed against the protein receptors on the membranes of neurons. These include N-methyl-D-aspartate receptor (NMDAR), voltage-gated potassium channel (VGKC)-complex, glutamic acid decarboxylase (GAD), and anti-contactin-associated protein-like 2 (CASPR2) antibody autoantibodies. Autoimmune encephalitis should be considered when the onset of epilepsy is relatively abrupt, seizures are not well controlled on antiepileptic drugs, and other problems affecting brain function also emerge over the same period. Some of these disorders respond very well to therapies that decrease immune system activity, such as intravenous gamma globulin and steroids.

HEREDITARY INFLUENCES AND EPILEPSY: WHAT ARE THE CHANCES?

Hereditary (genetic) factors play a larger role in generalized than focal epilepsy. What does this mean for other members of the family? Among children with generalized epilepsy and generalized spike-waves on the EEG, the risk of epilepsy in a sibling is approximately 4 percent. When a child with absence or tonic–clonic seizures has generalized spikes and waves and one of that child's brothers or sisters also has the spike-wave abnormality, another child in the family has an 8 percent risk of developing epilepsy. When a parent and a child have generalized epilepsy, there is a 10 percent risk that the parent's other children will have isolated seizures or epilepsy.

Heredity may also influence the likelihood that a person will develop focal epilepsy after experiencing a cause of seizures, such as severe head injury. The rate of epilepsy is higher among family members of people who develop epilepsy with cerebral palsy than among the relatives of people who do not. Benign rolandic epilepsy and several others (see Chapter 3) are partial epilepsy syndromes with a genetic component.

The children of parents with epilepsy also have an increased risk, but that risk may be lower than one might expect. By age 25 years, a child of a parent with epilepsy has a 6 percent chance of having an unprovoked seizure, compared with 1 to 2 percent in the general population. Epilepsy is more common among the children of women with epilepsy than among the children of men with epilepsy. With a person who developed epilepsy at a young age, there is an increased risk that that person's siblings and children will have epilepsy.

In cases where heredity is important, a single gene or several genes may be the determining factor. More than 90 epilepsy genes are known, and new ones are identified each year. However, most of these genetic disorders are uncommon or rare.

Parents first encounter epilepsy as an isolated seizure. As you begin to learn your child's epilepsy—the syndrome and possible causes—your child's epilepsy gains context. You will better understand where your child fits into the greater epilepsy picture and can start to chart a path for your child's next step.

II | DIAGNOSIS AND TREATMENT OF EPILEPSY

The first step to controlling your child's epilepsy is diagnosis: working with your doctor and medical team to identify your child's seizure type and syndrome—and confirming that the seizures are, in fact, epilepsy. With a diagnosis in hand, it's time to consider possible treatments, if necessary. Treatments fall into three main categories: medications, diets, and surgery and devices. Diagnosis and treatment can involve some trial and error, as all children are different and all epilepsies are different.

5 THE FIRST AND SECOND SEIZURES: DIAGNOSING EPILEPSY

THE FIRST SEIZURE

Daniel had just gotten to the breakfast table; I was rushing around getting ready for his first day of camp. Suddenly, his sister yelled, "Mom!" Daniel's eyes looked frozen; he fell to the floor and started shaking his arms and legs. I told his sister to call 911 and ran to his side; he was sleeping by the time EMS arrived. When they asked me how long the seizure was, I told them it felt like forever. Daniel is a healthy kid. Why did this happen? ■ ■ ■

Your child's first seizure almost certainly came as a surprise to you, one that can set off an array of emotions, from confusion to fear. The child himself usually won't remember the seizure, which means that the episode ends up being most frightening for the family members and other witnesses. And then, once the shock wears off, the overwhelming questions set in. Why did this happen? Will he have another one? Does he need to take medication? If so, will he have to take the medication for the rest of his life? The simplest way to deal with the questions and begin calming the fear is through education—not just about the medical aspect of epilepsy, but also about the social and psychological impacts on the child and the family. (See Part III for further exploration of this impact.)

After a child's first seizure, no matter how mild, he should be evaluated by a doctor to rule out any underlying causes. This first evaluation includes someone taking a careful detailed history of the event and of the child's recent history (illness, sleep deprivation, etc.), a comprehensive physical examination, blood tests, and often an MRI (a CT scan be valuable in the emergency room, but an MRI is preferred outside that setting). Most single seizures do not result from a clearly defined cause, such as a structural abnormality that would show up on an MRI. Still, the neuroimaging is important because it can rule out potential life-threatening, although extremely uncommon, causes such as brain tumors, strokes, or serious infection. When, as usually happens, the results of these tests are normal or reveal a benign cause of the seizure, the child is typically sent home from the emergency room or doctor's office—often with a prescription for a rescue medication that can be used at home in case of a recurrent seizure that lasts more than three to five minutes.

THE FIRST OFFICE EVALUATION

The Patient's History

After being evaluated in the emergency room, all tests came back negative and we were discharged to go home. Daniel seems to be back to his usual self, but I can't help but worry—what if he has another seizure? ▪ ▪ ▪

After life-threatening underlying causes are ruled out in the emergency room, it's time for a more in-depth evaluation in a doctor's office. During the first office visit, the doctor will begin by asking the main reason or chief complaint for the visit and then will ask more detailed questions pertaining to your child's symptoms. A significant portion of the exam will be devoted to the taking of a full medical history. This is an important exchange between you and the medical team to help paint a full picture of who your child is and any relevant information (for example, sleep deprivation) that may explain why the seizure occurred. The doctor will start with your child's prenatal and birth history and lead up to the current day, highlighting any pertinent data. (Note: Unless your child has cerebral palsy, there is no association between birth history and epilepsy.) You or your child, depending on age, will be asked a series of questions directly related to the seizure. (Prior to your appointment, if possible, be sure to send in any medical records that you already have in hand, such as notes from other doctors, results of laboratory studies, and electroencephalography [EEG] and MRI reports and CDs.)

This medical history serves as the foundation for diagnosing epilepsy. Because most doctors infrequently witness a patient's actual seizure in person, this discussion gives your doctor the chance to gather the pertinent details. You may be asked the following questions:

Before the seizure:

▪ Was your child lacking sleep or feeling unusual stress?

▪ Did he experience any recent illness?

▪ Had your child or adolescent taken any medications or drugs, including over-the-counter drugs (such as cold medications), alcohol, or illegal drugs?

▪ What was he doing immediately before the seizure: lying, sitting, standing, getting up from a lying position, heavy exercise?

During the seizure:

▪ What time of day did it occur?

▪ Did it occur around the transition into or out of sleep?

- How did it begin?
- Was there any warning just prior to the seizure's onset?
- Did he exhibit any abnormal movements of the eyes, mouth, face, head, arms, or legs during the episode?
- Was he able to talk and respond appropriately?
- Was there loss of urine or feces?
- Did he bite his tongue or the inside of his cheeks?

After the seizure:

- Was your child confused or tired?
- Was your child's speech normal?
- Did he have a headache?
- Was any part of his body weak?
- How long did it take for him to fully recover?

Because an accurate description from an eyewitness is invaluable, it may be helpful to write your own brief summary of the seizure prior to the appointment. This can be tough to do—experiencing your child having a seizure can be very upsetting and disorienting—but taking the time to consider all the information before your appointment ensures that the doctor will get the most accurate information as he makes assessments and considers treatment options. If you were not present during the episode, ask any witnesses to either write down detailed descriptions before their memories fade, to come to the doctor's office with you, or to speak with the doctor/nurse separately about their observations. Save these witnesses' notes after the initial appointment; they can be helpful if you see other doctors in the future. If the seizures recur, try to capture them on home video, either with your phone or another device.

You should also review your greater family history, either before or soon after the office visit. Did other family members have seizures with fever in infancy or early childhood? Has anyone else in the family had epilepsy or other neurological disorders, disorders associated with loss of consciousness, or any symptoms similar to those of the child? Did your child incur a head injury during his birth, one that involved loss of consciousness? If yes, how long was the loss of consciousness? Has your child ever had meningitis (infection of the membranes around the brain and spinal cord) or encephalitis (viral infection of the brain)?

If your child has had more than one episode of seizures, try to identify factors that were similar each time. For example, some adolescent girls with epilepsy have more frequent seizures just before or during menstruation. Or perhaps you've noted that your child was under significant stress right before his seizures. Sometimes these kinds of specific environmental factors (such as sleep deprivation, antibiotic use, heat, and fluorescent lights) can have an effect on your child's episodes, so you'll want to bring them up to your doctor.

Be aware, however, that these associations between environmental factors and seizures are also often coincidental. By carefully documenting when the possible factor occurs in relation to when the seizures happen, you can help your medical team establish whether there is an actual association between the two.

It is not uncommon to have a lot of questions during your first visit. Many parents find it helpful to bring a list of questions with them to the doctor's office. These questions are best asked at the end of the visit, after the doctor has heard the history, reviewed medical records, and examined your child. Try to focus the questions during this initial appointment. Your dialogue with your doctor and learning about epilepsy and your child's condition will evolve. Often, you will meet with members of the nursing staff who will be able to answer more of your questions and provide reading materials. Also consider consulting online resources such as epilepsy.com and reaching out to your local Epilepsy Foundation or hospital support resources of patient groups.

The General Medical Examination

Seizures can result from some medical disorders, which is why a general medical examination is part of the first consultation. Among the disorders that may cause seizures are abnormalities of the skin and brain such as neurocutaneous syndromes (including tuberous sclerosis complex, neurofibromatosis, and Sturge–Weber syndrome). Identification of characteristic skin findings can diagnosis these syndromes. If indicated, an examination and laboratory studies can assess the functioning of the liver, kidneys, and other organ systems to rule out illnesses such as hyperthyroidism. If a medical disorder or syndrome other than epilepsy is detected and medication is recommended, the interactions between this medication and any medications prescribed to treat the seizures must be considered.

The Neurological Examination

The next step for many children who've had seizures is a neurological exam by a pediatric neurologist to assess the function of your child's brain, spinal cord, nerves, and muscles. To be more specific, the neurologist looks at mental functions, such as your child's ability to maintain eye contact, pay attention, name objects, and remember words, and then systematically evaluates your child's strength, sensation, reflexes, coordination, walking, and other functions.

In additional to this initial evaluation, doctors often do brief screening examinations during follow-up visits to identify any changes in the child's neurological function. If the child has increasingly impaired concentration, slow or slurred speech, unsteady walking, jerking eye movements when his eyes are directed toward one side, or trembling when his arms are outstretched, for example, the doctor may need to reduce the medication dose. These follow-up exams vary in time, but for patients without other problems such as developmental delays or behavioral problems, the visit may be brief, especially if the patient has no new complaints.

Diagnostic Testing

The neurologist will likely request a diagnostic test or tests to gain more information about your child's health. Depending on your child's history, the doctor may ask for an EEG scan and/or a neuroimaging test, which are discussed in this section.

THE ELECTROENCEPHALOGRAPHY

Electroencephalography (EEG), a painless procedure that records the brain's activity, is the most specific test for diagnosing epilepsy. Unfortunately, many young and developmentally disabled children find the experience of having the EEG electrodes placed stressful and unpleasant, which makes it difficult for their parents as well. Bringing your child's favorite music or video may help distract them and make them more comfortable. For babies, it is helpful to perform the EEG around naptime. You'll likely be able to be with your child while the electrodes are applied, and some testing centers may allow you to lie with the child during the test administration. If your child is still an infant, a bottle may help to calm him beforehand, and then the baby can sleep naturally during the test itself. Sedation is rarely needed for some children with autism or other behavioral disorders.

Before the test, electrodes are applied to a patient's scalp and connected by wires to an electrical box, which in turn is connected to an EEG machine (Figure 5.1A). The technologist may measure the child's head so that the electrodes—small metal cup-shaped disks—can be placed in the correct position. To improve the quality of the recording, the technologist may also use a mildly abrasive cream to scrub each position before applying the electrodes with a conductive paste. Some labs use EEG caps that can be rapidly applied, but these may have limitations. During the test itself, the EEG digitally records the patient's brain waves as a series of squiggly lines (Figure 5.1B). Each trace corresponds to a different region of the brain. The EEG does not stimulate the head with electricity and poses no danger.

A completed EEG scan shows the patterns of normal and/or abnormal electrical activity within a patient's brain. Abnormal patterns may be either nonspecific or specific. Nonspecific patterns are characteristic in many different conditions. For example, slow nonspecific waves may occur after head trauma, a stroke, brain tumor, migraine, or seizures. Slow waves have a lower frequency (cycles per second or Hertz) than would be typical for a normal person

FIGURE 5.1A: A patient being set up with electrodes attached to an EEG machine.

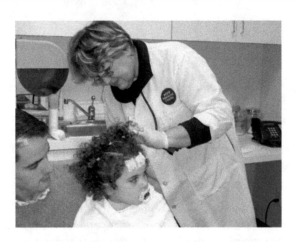

FIGURE 5.1B: EEG traces from a person without epilepsy, at rest. Each line corresponds to an area of the brain from which the EEG recording was made.

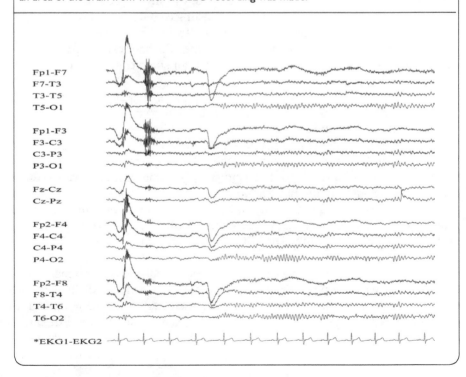

of the patient's age. Spikes, sharp waves, and spike-and-wave discharges are considered specific patterns that indicate a tendency toward seizures. Spikes and sharp waves occurring in a local area of the brain, such as the left temporal lobe, are seen in patients with focal epilepsy (Figure 5.2). Spike-and-wave discharges beginning simultaneously over both hemispheres are markers of generalized epilepsy (Figure 5.3). In some cases, seizures are recorded during the EEG, particularly in children who experience absence seizures during increased breathing (hyperventilation).

Because the EEG usually records brain activity between seizures, which is called interictal activity (*ictal* means seizure-related), EEG results for a child with epilepsy taken during a random 30-minute sampling are often completely normal. Remember that seizures occupy a tiny percentage of a child's life, so the EEG can be normal for many epilepsy patients. Also, areas of abnormality may remain undetected by the EEG if the activity arises from deep regions "outside the reach" of the scalp electrodes or if the volume of brain affected is too small to

FIGURE 5.2: EEG traces of spikes and sharp waves (epilepsy waves) from the left temporal lobe (rows 1–4) of a person with focal epilepsy. The traces from the right frontal and temporal lobes (rows 5–8) are normal.

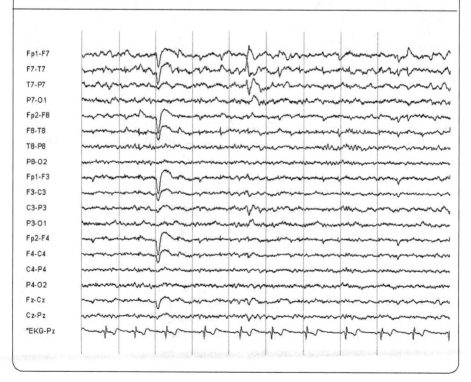

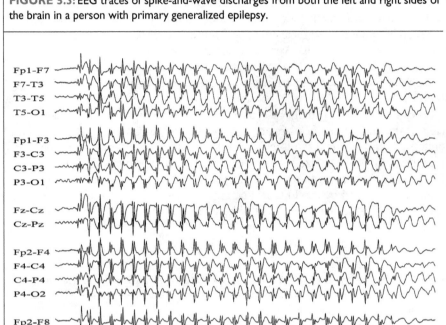

FIGURE 5.3: EEG traces of spike-and-wave discharges from both the left and right sides of the brain in a person with primary generalized epilepsy.

generate abnormal waves of sufficient size. The chance of finding an abnormality on the EEG is increased if the test is recorded in the following circumstances:

- During both wakefulness and sleep
- After sleep deprivation
- With three to five minutes of deep breathing (hyperventilation)
- With flashing lights (photic stimulation)
- With additional electrodes
- For prolonged periods

The initial recording typically lasts only 20 to 40 minutes, and the same amount of time is generally needed to prepare for it. Thus, the EEG procedure usually takes 60 to 90 minutes of the patient's time. The test is performed by an EEG technologist (see Chapter 8). The patient can help by washing his hair the night before or the day of the test, but should avoid using conditioners, hair creams, sprays, or styling gels.

AMBULATORY EEG

A brain's electrical activity fluctuates from second to second. As a result, an extended recording featuring long periods of wakefulness and sleep is more likely to capture electrical abnormalities than a 20- to 40-minute routine EEG, and this type of recording may be ordered for your child if the initial EEG findings are not specific enough. The test is done by an ambulatory EEG device that can record 24 to 72 hours of information while the patient goes about most of his usual activities. (Video recording capacity may also be available to accompany these readings.) The ambulatory EEG recorder fits in a small carrying case, with the wires running either under or outside of the patient's shirt (Figure 5.4). Most children prefer not to go to school while attached to the device, and because the electrodes must stay on the head for a longer time than for a routine EEG, a type of glue is often used. Still, the test comes with little or no discomfort, and the technologist can easily remove this glue with acetone or a similar solution once the recording is complete. If removing the leads at home, gentle shampooing and a fine-toothed comb should remove the glue.

While a child is attached to the ambulatory EEG, parents (or the child himself, if an adolescent) should keep a diary of activities. Most recorders have an "event"

FIGURE 5.4: Recording the 24-hour ambulatory EEG. The device records the EEG signals from the electrodes on the patient's scalp while she pursues daily activities.

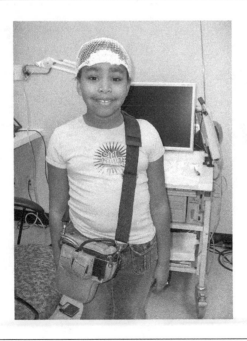

button for children or family members to press if typical seizure symptoms occur, such as episodes of feeling "spacey" or confused.

In general, medications are not lowered or stopped during ambulatory EEGs, and any changes should be discussed with your child's doctor. It is often helpful to have the child engage in normal activities, especially those that are associated with behaviors that are suspected of being possible seizure triggers.

VIDEO-EEG MONITORING

Video-EEG monitoring allows prolonged recording of the patient's behavior (audio and video) alongside EEG readings, which can be viewed on a split screen. This permits a precise correlation of brain electrical activity and behavior during the episodes (Figure 5.5). During video-EEG recordings, electrodes are usually glued to the scalp with collodion. Video-EEG results can help determine whether a patient's episodes are epileptic seizures, and if so, the type of seizures and the region of the brain from which the seizures originate.

FIGURE 5.5: Video-EEG monitoring. (A) A patient being monitored; a video camera (not shown) records her activities, including any seizures that occur, and the EEG signals from the electrodes on her head are transmitted to an adjoining monitor. (B) The patient's seizures and EEG are recorded simultaneously and shown as a split-screen display on a television monitor.

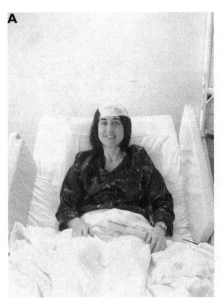
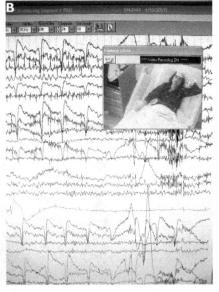

Video-EEG recordings can be done on hospitalized inpatients or on outpatients. The advantage of inpatient monitoring is that it allows the physician to closely monitor the patient and adjust medications or other factors during the test. Medication reduction, sleep deprivation, hyperventilation, or exercise may be used to induce seizures so that they can be recorded on the device.

A child who is going to have inpatient video-EEG monitoring should bring clothing to the hospital that can be buttoned up, not pullovers. And please do not forget to bring video games, movies, games, and reading materials, and things to keep him entertained. A hospital stay can be boring for your child and yourselves.

NEUROIMAGING OF THE BRAIN

Neuroimaging provides pictures of the brain. The neuroimaging test most commonly used to assess children with epilepsy is an MRI of the head. MRI scans help determine whether an abnormality in the structure of the brain—such as excess spinal fluid (hydrocephalus), scar tissue, or a tangle of blood vessels (vascular malformation)—may be causing a child's epilepsy. An MRI is strongly preferred over a CT scan because it provides much more information and does not use x-rays. In emergency room settings, however, a CT is often the only available test and can identify disorders that require urgent treatment.

The MRI is usually called for after a child has had one or more seizures, in order to see if a structural (physical) cause is present. For most children with focal seizures especially, an MRI should be obtained to look for abnormalities. Even if the cause of a child's seizures is known, a repeat MRI scan will likely be considered if that cause is one that can evolve or change over time (for example, a benign tumor or a vascular (blood vessel) malformation) or if the clinical picture changes significantly. An MRI is often not needed, however, for children with well-defined epilepsy syndromes that are generalized (and presumably genetic), such as absence seizures or juvenile myoclonic epilepsy, as well as benign rolandic epilepsy. The MRI results in these cases are almost always normal or unrelated to epilepsy.

Magnetic Resonance Imaging

An MRI provides detailed images of the brain's structure (Figure 5.6). The machine that performs MRIs does not use x-rays, but rather uses a powerful magnet that changes the spin on atomic particles and then measures the changes in the magnetic field as the particles resume their previous course. MRIs can identify small areas of scar tissue, abnormal brain development (dysplasia), tumors, and other problems.

The MRI is safe and painless. Some children naturally become frightened at first when they see or experience the confined space in which the MRI is taken. You can lessen this by talking with your child before the test about how it is performed and warning him about the machine's loud noises, whose effects can

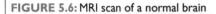

FIGURE 5.6: MRI scan of a normal brain

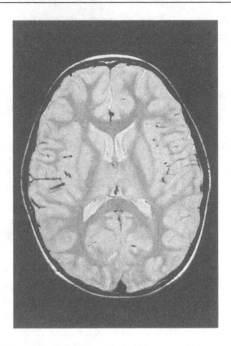

be reduced with earplugs, and by allowing your child to listen to music. Young children often require sedation before the test, and medications for relaxation can be given to older children if they require it. In addition, a less-confined MRI machine (open MRI) can be used, although open MRIs provide less detail than is ideal for many patients.

Related scanning techniques include the functional MRI (fMRI), positron emission tomography (PET), and single photon emission spectroscopy (SPECT scan), all highly specialized tests that are not part of an initial workup following a seizure. If seizures continue despite medication or if there is a strong suspicion of seizure source requiring surgery (see Chapter 14), these tests may be indicated.

WHAT IS THE RISK OF SEIZURE RECURRENCE?

Half of all children with no other medical history who suffer a single, unprovoked convulsive seizure won't have a second seizure. These children will need no treatment and usually have no lingering effects from the episode. With children who do have another episode, that second episode almost always comes within two years; most occur within six months. If a child has had two seizures, the risk of a third is about 80 percent. Children with brain injuries (head trauma, infection, or other type of brain abnormality, leading to a diagnosis of symptomatic epilepsy) or an abnormal neurological examination are at higher risk for seizure recurrence than those with no risk factors (epilepsies with no known cause). A history of an abnormal EEG also places a child at higher risk of recurrence.

THE SECOND SEIZURE...TO TREAT OR NOT TO TREAT?

Two weeks after his first seizure, Daniel was getting ready to go to bed and he had a second seizure. Daniel recovered and the following morning was asking to go to camp. Our pediatrician recommended we bring Daniel to an epilepsy doctor. Daniel's office examination was normal and she recommended medication but wanted a prolonged EEG study to see if it helped guide medication choice and better understand his disorder. I don't want Daniel to have any more seizures, but I am worried about having to give him medicine every day. ▪ ▪ ▪

Once a child has had a second seizure, it's time to meet with your doctor to discuss treatment options, including antiepileptic medication. The goal is for your child to have no further seizures. In considering medication, the doctor will look at your child's current state of health and well-being, the probable frequency of his seizures if untreated, and the medication's possible side effects. Children with absence seizures, complex partial seizures, myoclonic seizures, or infantile spasms will usually have recurrences, and medication is often indicated in these cases. An exception is benign epilepsy of childhood, where a child may have a tonic–clonic seizure, yet medication is not often necessary (see Seizure Types and Syndromes, Chapters 3 and 4). A child with a single tonic–clonic seizure, normal neurological exam, normal MRI, and normal EEG with no other risk factors is generally not started on medication. Treatment is often recommended for a child who has had two or more tonic–clonic seizures. All of this should be discussed in detail with the physician treating your child.

The aim in choosing medications is to achieve seizure freedom for your child with the minimum dosage and the fewest side effects (for more on medications, see Chapters 9 and 10). You should talk with your child's health care team about any suspected side effects that occur after medication is begun. In many cases, if the side effects are expected and mild (such as stomach discomfort or dizziness), they'll often resolve within a week or two. If a child experiences troublesome side effects that don't resolve, speaking with the child's health care team and switching to another medication (one that may be without side effects, or with lesser effects) is typically recommended. Parents are excellent resources when it comes to recognizing small changes in their children. Have confidence in yourself as a caregiver. Family-centered care—care involving family members as careful observers who work collaboratively with the child's health care team— maximizes the potential for successful treatment.

Obtaining maximum seizure control and limiting side effects is both a science and an art that will vary by doctor, child, and medication. The goal is to find a balance that allows your child to have the best quality of life possible. Sometimes reducing or changing your child's drug may increase seizures but be worth it in terms of how that change improves his quality of life. For example, two minutes a month of mild seizure activity with few to no side effects is often better for children than no seizures at the expense of feeling tired all day long.

Parents should never adjust their child's medication without approval from the doctor. If a medication is prescribed that's not covered by your insurance, if the child is experiencing side effects, or if any other problems occur, be sure to notify your child's doctor. Sometimes a little bit of knowledge is a dangerous thing. For example, a very well educated parent read about a drug's potential side effect and noted that her child was more tired, so she lowered one medication by half to compensate. The result was a prolonged and dangerous seizure. The side effect did not occur in her child and the dramatic reduction in a key medication was catastrophic.

Because children who have had a second seizure are likely to have a third, it is important during this visit, if not during the first, to discuss with your doctor a plan in case of any further breakthrough seizures. This will allow you as a parent to be prepared and can prevent unnecessary emergency room visits for your child.

FIRST AID FOR SEIZURES

My younger sister Meghan was just diagnosed with seizures. We often go to the movies, shopping trips, and runs at our local park. The doctor gave her medicine for her seizures, but I am afraid I won't know what to do should she have a seizure when we are together. What should I do if Meghan has a seizure? ■ ■ ■

Witnessing someone who has a seizure can be frightening, especially if that person is a loved one. Yet a calm approach and basic first aid knowledge on the part of the witnesses can minimize potential complications (Table 5.1). So for people who have family members with epilepsy, knowledge of how to respond to a seizure is important. Siblings like the teenager in the preceding vignette should be educated about epilepsy and even first aid when they have the maturity to understand and help.

Tonic–clonic seizures especially appear life threatening, with their sudden onset, falls, and convulsive movements, but they are almost always self-limited and do not cause serious problems. During the seizure, the child should be placed on his side and protected from his environment. Do not try to put anything in the child's mouth; he will not swallow his tongue. Do not restrain the child's movement.

Most seizures stop on their own within five minutes. A rescue medication will also likely be prescribed, which you, as the parent, can administer in the

TABLE 5.1: BASIC FIRST AID DURING SEIZURE ACTIVITY

- Protect from injury
- If wearing scarf of multiple layers of clothes, loosen around face and neck
- DO NOT PLACE ANYTHING IN CHILD'S MOUTH
- If child is walking or sitting in chair, place an arm around child's shoulder to provide stability so that injury is avoided
- If able to, lay flat and place on side; do not restrain
- Speak to child in reassuring tone that all is okay and that he/she is okay
- Stay with child at all times
- Use watch to time the duration of the seizure

If rescue medication has been prescribed, administer as indicated.

If at any moment, there is concern for the child's safety, respiratory effort (spontaneous breathing), or seizure continues despite intervention, EMS (911) should be activated.

event of a breakthrough seizure lasting longer than three to five minutes. For children with a history of prolonged seizures, rescue medication can be given at seizure onset. There are different forms of rescue medication, and the child's age and seizure type are taken into consideration when choosing which one is appropriate for your family. The most commonly used rescue medications are rectal diazepam (Diastat), nasal midazolam, buccal (between gum and cheek) midazolam, and dissolvable clonazepam wafers or clonazepam or lorazepam tablets. If the seizure lasts longer than five minutes and no rescue medication is available, or the seizure lasts more than three to five minutes after rescue medication is administered, EMS should be called so the child can be evaluated. For more on first aid and epilepsy, see Chapter 10 and Appendix B, as well as http://www.epilepsy.com/get-help/seizure-first-aid.

FOLLOW-UP VISITS

Once a treatment plan is in place, you'll continue to touch base with the pediatric neurologist or epileptologist treating your child's epilepsy to make sure the treatment is on track, make adjustments as needed, and share any information that may influence the treatment or the doctor's initial diagnosis. These follow-up appointments typically last between 15 and 30 minutes. If your child is seizure-free and tolerating the medication prescribed, the visit may be brief. If the seizures are ongoing, increased in frequency, or your child is experiencing side effects from the medication, the visit will have to be longer. When there is a need to discuss more complex subjects, such as the possibility of considering epilepsy surgery or discontinuing medication, a longer appointment may be required. Let your doctor's office know when scheduling the appointment if you think additional time might be necessary.

It's important during these visits to let the doctor know exactly how the epilepsy is affecting your child and family, so that the medical team to be able to best care for all of you. Even with all of this information, there's sometimes a gap between how a doctor perceives a child is doing and how the child and/or parents feel he is doing. Be honest and open with your child's physician regarding any health concerns in order to ensure proper care for your child.

Your child's first seizure may be a one-time occurrence, or it may be the start of an ongoing disorder. Either way, armed with research and with the help of an experienced medical team, you are your child's greatest advocate. It's up to you to observe your child's seizures and reactions to medication and to relay this information to the medical team. Seizure diaries are very helpful and simple to keep. Seizure diaries can help you and your doctor identify patterns (time of day, precipitating factors, cycles of seizure occurrence, etc.). There are two very good free apps for seizure diaries (http://www.epilepsy.com/get-help/my-epilepsy-diary and https://www.seizuretracker.com). You are also, to your child, the most familiar face as you move through the medical visits and beyond. By carefully explaining what the visits and tests will entail, you can help demystify experiences that to a child (and often a parent) can at first seem confusing and possibly scary.

6 | IS IT EPILEPSY? DISORDERS AND BEHAVIORS THAT MIMIC EPILEPSY

It's easy to think when your child has a seizure that it's a symptom of epilepsy, but often that's not the case. Most of the time when a person experiences shakes, jerks, or staring spells, she is not actually having a seizure and does not have epilepsy. So, how do you determine if these types of sudden changes in behavior are the result of normal activity, of seizures—or of another disorder? As we discussed in Chapter 5, a diagnosis of epilepsy is based on the history but can be supported with test results such as electroencephalogram (EEG), MRI, but sometimes it can be difficult, since many other disorders cause symptoms that mimic those of a seizure. It's not unusual in those first office visits for doctors—as well as parents searching the Internet—to jump to a diagnosis and then work to make the evidence fit that diagnosis. Yet initial diagnoses can be incorrect.

This is again why your input as a parent is vital. In all medical diagnoses, the history taken from the patient and observers is the most important element. Though diagnostic MRIs and EEGs, as well as prolonged EEG recordings, can make and confirm epilepsy diagnoses, their readings can't replace the vital information gleaned from an accurate description of the events that occurred before, during, and after a patient's episode. The witnesses—as well as the child if she is able—should give the doctor as much information as possible about the event. If certain details are vague, the doctor should be told that they are vague. If a video is available from a phone or other device, these are often very helpful, especially in the case of recurrent events. It's important to remember, though, that no matter how accurate and complete the information, and even if the entire event is captured on video, some episodes remain difficult for experts to diagnose. Every epilepsy specialist has had patients for whom the initial diagnosis was incorrect. Doctors might be convinced they've witnessed one particular disorder after seeing an episode in their office, only to have subsequent evidence confirm another. This is one reason that follow-up care and the additional information it provides are essential.

DIAGNOSIS OF NEWBORN AND INFANT SEIZURES

In determining whether a newborn or infant's seizures are a symptom of epilepsy, the doctor will take into account the child's medical history and physical examination, and may order tests to look for:

- Structural abnormalities in the brain, using an ultrasound, CT scan, or MRI

- Abnormal electrical activity in the brain, using an EEG

- Metabolic problems, using tests of the blood, urine, and possibly spinal fluid

- Genetic disorders, using chromosomal and DNA studies

- Evidence of infection or metabolic disorders, using a spinal tap (lumbar puncture)

The lumbar puncture is a safe procedure that provides a sample of spinal fluid. The procedure is mildly painful; in fact, the baby's worst crying during this test may come when the doctor cleans the skin with a cool antiseptic solution. An anesthetic cream can be used on the skin just prior to the test, and anesthesia is sometimes administered as well.

Rarely, seizures in newborns and infants result from a vitamin B6 (pyridoxine) deficiency, which is very treatable. The diagnosis can be established by recording the EEG while injecting vitamin B6. An improvement in the EEG patterns after the injection indicates a vitamin B6 deficiency.

In many cases, no cause can be found. Brain malformations that cause seizures may be impossible to pinpoint, especially injuries that occurred in the womb or those associated with only microscopic damage.

Diagnostic Challenges by Age

Newborns. Seizures in newborns (in the first month of life) can be difficult for even experts to recognize. One reason is that seizures in newborns may appear as fragments of the kinds of seizures you'd see in older children. For example, the infant's brain is still developing and often cannot make the coordinated responses characteristic of a tonic–clonic seizure. The baby may have jerking or stiffening of a leg or an arm that alternates from side to side, or the whole upper body may suddenly jerk forward, or both legs may jerk up toward the belly with the knees bent. The baby's facial expression, breathing, and heart rate may change. In addition, impairment of responsiveness, which is critical in defining many types of seizures in children and adults, is difficult to assess in newborns. Parents may suspect that awareness is impaired when the child does not respond to their voice or when the luster in the child's eyes is replaced by a glaze.

Neurologists are often told not to watch their own babies or young children too closely, especially when they sleep, because normal movements sometimes mimic fragments of seizures or other disorders. Normal babies exhibit many sudden and brief jerks, grimaces, stares, and mouth movements that might suggest seizures. The likelihood that these behavioral changes are a seizure increases if the changes are repetitive and identical in their features and duration, if the episodes are not brought on by changes in posture or activity such as eating, and if the behaviors are not typical of children of the same age. It's helpful to videotape the suspected behavior for a doctor to review—but, as mentioned earlier, looks can deceive even expert eyes.

One behavior in babies that's easily mistaken for a seizure is the Moro or startle reflex. When a baby is startled (such as by momentary removal of support of its head, a loud noise, or a bright light), its spine will stiffen, its arms and legs extend outward from its body, and its fingers fan out. This is called the Moro reflex. It is present in its full form until a child is three months old, and remains in an incomplete form until five months. Another normal infant behavior is jitters or shivering movements or tremors that are similar to the shivering that occurs with fever in older children and adults. Normal newborns also display repetitive sucking movements of the mouth and jerks during sleep—sleep myoclonus is often confused with seizures.

A rare genetic disorder known as benign familial neonatal seizures (BFNS) can also be responsible for an infant's seizures. Infants with BFNS experience frequent brief seizures beginning around day three of life. The disorder usually is inherited by an autosomal dominant gene (that is, one parent also had the disorder), but it may also result from a spontaneous mutation in the child's DNA. The seizures usually stop by five months of age. Some BFNS cases result from a potassium-channel gene mutation that can also be responsible for a much more serious epilepsy that first arises in infancy and is associated with developmental delays. Other rare genetic disorders that cause seizures in newborn babies include glucose transporter protein 1 (GLUT1) deficiency syndrome (due to a defect in the SLC2A1 gene), which may respond well to the ketogenic diet (see Chapter 11).

An EEG is very helpful in defining seizures in newborns but can be more difficult to interpret than in older children.

Infants. Seizures in infants (babies from 1 to 12 months old) appear similar to those in newborns. Because older infants can focus their attention briefly, parents and doctors are better able to identify impaired consciousness during these children's seizures. Yet seizures cannot be diagnosed entirely from observing a child who has a fixed stare, since normal children daydream and it may be difficult to distract even the healthiest of babies at times. Other nonepileptic mimics of epilepsy in infants include gastroesophageal reflux (GERD), a common disorder in children that can cause a diverse range of symptoms, including vomiting, coughing, and eating difficulties. In some babies, GERD can trigger sudden jerking movements that mimic myoclonic seizures and infantile spasms. The diagnosis is more challenging in young children who cannot describe their symptoms. Other metabolic or hormonal disorders can cause behavioral changes that may be mistaken for seizures. *Febrile seizures* are usually tonic–clonic seizures that may occur in infants and young children when they have a high fever or illness (see Chapter 3).

Nearly all seizures in infants, regardless of cause, last less than five minutes. If seizures last more than five minutes or occur in a series, the baby should be taken to an emergency room unless a specific therapy and plan were previously discussed with the doctor.

CONDITIONS CONFUSED WITH EPILEPSY IN OLDER CHILDREN

In children older than one year, many medical, neurological, and psychiatric disorders can mimic seizures. These disorders should be considered when making a diagnosis of epilepsy, since launching into the correct course of treatment depends on having a correct diagnosis. Only the few disorders that are most often mistaken for epileptic seizures are presented here.

Fainting

> Sara came to the Epilepsy Center after having five episodes of dizziness followed by loss of consciousness, all over a period of six months. Witnesses said her arms jerked and her eyes "rolled up in her head" during the episodes; these witnesses assumed what they'd seen were seizures. The neurologist found that all five events happened when Sara was dehydrated or after experiencing pain. Sara underwent a prolonged EEG study that came back with normal results, and underwent a tilt-table test that showed her blood pressure dropping abnormally when she was in certain positions. Sara was reassured by her neurologist that she had neurogenic syncope—a fancy word for fainting—not epileptic seizures. ▪ ▪ ▪

Fainting (also known as syncope, meaning a brief loss of consciousness) is most often caused by the brain not receiving enough blood. Fainting is common and rarely serious. It usually happens when a child is standing and complains of some combination of dizziness, lightheadedness, stomach discomfort, and blurry vision; then, she turns pale, may sweat, and then falls with a brief loss of consciousness. Her body may stiffen slightly, and her arms or legs may jerk several times. A misdiagnosis of epilepsy may be made when the doctor hears that the child suddenly lost consciousness, fell down, and had jerking movements. In rare cases, a faint can evolve into a full-blown convulsive seizure. In most cases of fainting, though, consciousness is lost for less than 20 seconds and the person is alert 10 to 30 seconds later. Falling, it turns out, isn't just an effect of the faint—it's also a natural remedy for the faint. The reason faints happen most frequently when a person is standing is that faints tend to result from the heart's inability to pump blood up to the brain—and when a person is horizontal, blood flows more easily to the head.

Frequent episodes of fainting should be thoroughly investigated by a doctor, as these spells may be the result of a variety of disorders. One common cause is orthostatic hypotension—a drop in blood pressure when standing from a lying or sitting position, often as a result of dehydration from inadequate fluid intake, increased sweating, diarrhea, or vomiting, as well as prolonged standing in a hot environment. Another common cause of fainting is a painful or emotional stimulus (such as a needle prick or looking at a friend's broken bone). In rare cases, fainting results from a serious disturbance in the heart rhythm for which diagnosis and treatment can be lifesaving. For any child who faints in which there is a family history of sudden death or who faints during exercise or in association with an intense emotion or startle, an electrocardiogram and/or cardiology consultation should be obtained to exclude a serious heart rhythm disturbance.

In a classic nonepileptic *"blue" breath-holding spell,* a young child cries intensely for a brief time (usually after some minor upset such as a bump on the head, being scolded, or when a toy is taken away), stops breathing in expiration, and then loses consciousness (faints) and becomes limp. The child turns blue and, occasionally, may sweat profusely. The typical attack lasts 30 to 60 seconds. During more prolonged spells, the child's entire body may become rigid and jerk, as a lack of oxygen to the brain actually triggers a stiffening of the body that resembles an epileptic seizure, but is not; the child does not have epilepsy. The typical sequence of a physical or emotional upset, followed by crying and breath-holding, is key in diagnosis. The lack of oxygen in breath-holding spells and the occasional seizure that follows do not cause brain injury.

These breath-holding spells usually begin between six months and 18 months of age and stop before the child is six years old. About 25 percent of these patients have a family history of breath-holding spells. There is no treatment. Some parents report that distracting the child during his intense crying can prevent the spell, but this remains unproven.

Pallid infantile fainting is another disorder that may be confused with epilepsy, specifically with atonic, tonic, or tonic–clonic seizures. The child suddenly becomes pale (pallid) and then faints. Often family members have had similar spells in early childhood, sometimes called "pallid breath-holding spells." In contrast to breath-holding spells, these episodes are more often provoked by pain rather than crying. If the spells are prolonged, the child's entire body may become rigid and jerk as a result of the lack of oxygen to the brain. This disorder usually begins between 12 and 18 months of age and ends before age six. The prognosis is excellent for these children. Treatment is rarely needed.

Hypoglycemia

Hypoglycemia (low blood sugar) is a common physiological condition that often results from fasting in a young child (ketotic hypoglycemia). The child's stores of carbohydrates are depleted and then they burn fats for energy. Symptoms of hypoglycemia include irritability, sweating, fatigue, rapid breathing, dizziness, and fainting. Fruit juice or other carbohydrates will quickly reverse the problem. Serious forms of hypoglycemia are rare and can occur in diabetic children who take too much insulin or, even more rarely, who have an endocrine tumor of the pancreas.

Unfortunately, hypoglycemia is sometimes diagnosed (or misdiagnosed) without good evidence. The diagnosis should only be made when low blood-sugar levels are documented while typical symptoms occur and when sugar or carbohydrate consumption resolves the symptoms.

Sleep Attacks

In *sleep attacks*, a child has an irresistible urge to sleep and suddenly dozes off, usually for only minutes. Upon awakening, she feels refreshed. Sleep attacks may be a symptom of narcolepsy, a sleep disorder. These attacks usually occur during boring conditions. Children with narcolepsy may also suffer sudden loss of muscle tone causing them to drop things, nod their head, or fall when they experience strong emotions such as vigorous laughing or crying.

Sleep Apnea

Sleep apnea is a condition in which breathing is intermittently interrupted during sleep. Many children with sleep apnea snore. Their sleep is restless with frequent brief awakenings that the child is unaware of. The disrupted sleep can cause excessive daytime sleepiness, irritability, and impaired concentration and memory—the same way that nocturnal seizures can disrupt nighttime sleep and thereby affect performance the next day.

In a child with epilepsy, sleep apnea may worsen seizure control by impairing restful sleep.

Daydreaming

We all daydream, and children daydream more than adults. Daydreaming in children can easily be confused with absence or complex partial seizures, in which staring is a prominent and common feature. What separates these seizures from daydreaming are movements that include lip smacking, eye blinking, grimacing, or stiffening of muscle groups. All of these behaviors are common during seizures but not during daydreaming. Unlike seizures, daydreaming can be stopped by calling the child's name, producing a startling noise, tickling, saying something like, "Look at the kitty," or shutting off the TV. Absence and complex partial seizures are seldom stopped by such means, although the child may be partially responsive. Absence seizures usually last less than 10 seconds, and complex partial seizures tend to last 30 seconds to 3 minutes. Daydreaming often occurs when the child is tired or bored or is involved in monotonous activity, such as riding in a car; seizures can occur at any time. Seizures begin abruptly and often unnaturally (for example, in the middle of a sentence or playing with a toy), while daydreaming often is a continuation of a natural pause in activity such as reading.

Movement Disorders

Many movement disorders can be confused with tonic or motor seizures. Children with these disorders assume abnormal postures (parts of their body set in an unusual position, such as the fingers curled up as if in a cramp, or the foot turned inward) or make sudden, unusual movements (such as eye blinking or jerks of a body part), and the attacks may begin suddenly, thus mimicking seizures. Most of these movement disorders occur spontaneously, but others are follow specific events such as eating (Sandifer's syndrome due to reflux).

Tics are involuntary, repetitive, intermittent, brief movements; they are not seizures. Although tics are purposeless, they may resemble purposeful movements. The most common tics in children are eye blinks, facial grimaces, shoulder shrugs, and head movements. The most severe form is Tourette's syndrome, which is also associated with vocal tics ranging from grunts and throat-clearing sounds to involuntary cursing.

Sleep jerks (benign nocturnal myoclonus) are brief, involuntary muscular contractions that occur as a person falls asleep. In some cases, they may awaken someone who is drifting off to sleep. Sleep jerks are common in healthy children and adults but may be confused with myoclonic seizures.

Nonepileptic (Psychogenic) Seizures

Despite the use of two seizure medications, Madison, a nine-year-old girl, had frequent episodes of shaking and impaired responsiveness that often resolved after taking clonazepam, a drug that treats epilepsy and also panic disorders. An epilepsy specialist recorded several of Madison's episodes on video EEG and diagnosed nonepileptic seizures. It was found that she had been subjected to bullying by several girls at school and was too embarrassed to talk about this. With counseling, the episodes resolved and she came off of all medications. ■ ■ ■

Nonepileptic (psychogenic) seizures are attacks that resemble epileptic seizures but result from subconscious mental activity, not epileptic brain activity. Doctors consider most of these episodes psychological in nature, but not purposely produced. The person is usually unaware that the attacks are not "epileptic." Nonepileptic seizures are common, and some patients are incorrectly treated for epileptic seizures for years until the correct diagnosis is made. Nonepileptic seizures are most common in adolescents and adults, but they can also occur in young children. In adolescents and adults, they occur most often in females, though they affect both sexes equally in younger children. Some children with nonepileptic seizures also have epileptic seizures and require different treatments for each disorder.

Nonepileptic seizures can imitate almost any seizure type. Most often they resemble complex partial or tonic–clonic seizures. The degree of similarity varies considerably. Because doctors rarely witness an attack, their diagnoses are based on family members who report episodes in which the patient stares or stiffens and jerks. Certain features suggest that a seizure is nonepileptic:

- Wild movements such as thrashing or rolling from side to side

- Screaming, crying, and moaning

- Jerking or stiffening of all extremities, but with preserved consciousness

- Stiffening and jerking of the extremities with immediate resumption of normal alertness after the attack (tiredness or confusion typically occurs after a tonic–clonic seizure)

- Altered behavior that waxes and wanes (jerking or the inability to respond to questions comes and goes)

- Prolonged episodes, lasting longer than five minutes

No single one of these factors can definitively lead a doctor to diagnose a seizure as nonepileptic, since epileptic seizures may occasionally include one or more of these behaviors.

Nonepileptic seizures are usually diagnosed with video-EEG monitoring; approximately 5 percent of children referred to epilepsy centers for video-EEG turn out to have nonepileptic seizures. In others, the episodes are found to be another mimic of epilepsy, such as reflux. Doctors often try to have a family member observe the video-EEG-recorded attack to ensure that it resembles the usual episode.

The treatment of nonepileptic seizures varies depending on the underlying psychological issues. Sometimes, after the doctor tells the child that the attacks are psychological, the attacks stop. Coexisting depression or anxiety disorders may require medication. The prognosis for resolution of the disorder and for the patient's psychological well-being varies. Counseling or psychotherapy is often helpful. Among children (and adults) with nonepileptic seizures, a prior history of sexual abuse is more common than in the general population. This emotional trauma is considered the underlying stressor, although most children with nonepileptic seizures do not have a history of sexual abuse; in these children, other psychological stressors are likely responsible.

Panic Attacks

Panic attacks are episodes of profound fear and anxiety, often associated with increased heart and breathing rate, shortness of breath, sweating, nausea, chest discomfort, and other bodily and mental symptoms. Certain settings can bring on panic attacks. Doctors may incorrectly suspect that a person having a panic attack is suffering from a focal seizure if the child reports autonomic symptoms such as racing heart and stomach discomfort paired with intense fear. Unlike seizures, which begin suddenly and usually last less than three minutes, panic attacks often build up gradually and last longer than five minutes. Panic attacks can be treated with behavioral therapy and medications.

Ruling out these mimics as the cause of your child's seizures—or ruling out epilepsy, if one of these mimics is actually the cause—may happen on your first visit with the doctor, or may only happen later, as the doctor gets to know your child and her condition over time. You'll also interact with a number of other health professionals as your child goes through her initial examinations and diagnostic appointments, as detailed in Chapter 7. You should feel free sharing information and concerns with all of these professionals, many of whom will aid your doctor in various ways as he diagnoses, and sometimes reconsiders his diagnosis of, your child.

7 | THE HEALTH CARE TEAM

As you begin your child's medical care and throughout that care, you will meet many new faces, whether in your doctor's office at that initial visit, the hospital, or an epilepsy center. At times this can feel overwhelming, and it can be easy to forget that as a parent you are one of the most important members of the health care team. You know your child best, and the health care professionals your family meets will rely on you as the bridge to knowing how your child is responding to treatment, what side effects are being encountered, and other questions regarding your child's overall well-being. A collaborative partnership among parent, child, and health care team is as important as any treatment prescribed.

THE CORE TEAM

The Doctor and Patient/Parent

Your child's regular pediatrician should assess everyday health concerns. In some countries, she also serves the role of assessing and treating children with a range of neurological disorders, including epilepsy. In many regions, if seizures are suspected, a pediatric neurologist is consulted. Many parents also consult a pediatric neurologist (epileptologist) who specializes in caring for children with epilepsy. No matter the type of doctor, he or she and the patient/parents will have the same goals: no seizures, no side effects, and a great quality of life. You should feel comfortable communicating your child's symptoms and side effects, and any questions you have, to the doctor. Because the doctor sees your child for only a limited amount of time, she relies on the information relayed by you and your child, if the child is able to verbalize. This communication is essential not only in planning treatment, but also in developing a good relationship between the family and the doctor.

The doctor should use language you can understand when discussing why tests are being ordered, what is involved in the testing process, and both the risks and benefits of therapy. If you don't understand what you're being told about any element of treatment or your child's disorder, tell the doctor! As your child's advocate, you need to fully understand what is being discussed and any treatment options being offered. If your child is old enough to talk, he should be given the opportunity to ask questions. Your relationship with the doctor should be comfortable and based on trust.

For children with epilepsy that coexists with other health disorders such as diabetes, the specialists should communicate with each other and the pediatrician. It is ideal but by no means necessary for the doctors to be at the same medical center or practice. Communication is key—especially if the medications for the different disorders can interact or affect the other disorder. Ideally, the pediatrician receives input from all specialists and coordinates care, but in reality, the specialist who sees the child most frequently assumes a lead role in care. Parents should make sure the doctor's notes and lab results are sent to all doctors; this should always happen but all too often does not in our increasingly complex and fragmentary medical world.

The Nurse Practitioner

A nurse practitioner is a licensed practitioner with an advanced master's degree in a specialty such as pediatrics. He or she is able to practice both independently and in collaboration with an attending physician. You may meet with the nurse practitioner first, who may take a complete medical history and examine your child. The nurse practitioner can order and interpret tests, can diagnose and treat patients, and can prescribe medications including narcotics and other restricted substances.

Nurses

Nurses are very active in pediatric care. They may participate in the visit and review tests that have been ordered and explain the medication plan. The nurses on your child's team will be able to review any questions you have following the initial meeting with the physician, as well as provide written instructions and educational material. In many medical offices, the nurses take patient calls and will answer questions over the phone and in person. The nurses often spend more time with the patient than the physician, and parents should feel as comfortable speaking with the nurses as they do with the doctor. The nurses are often at the frontline, acting as liaisons between the patient and physician. Some parents insist on speaking exclusively to the doctor. While this is reasonable when it comes to big decisions, parents who aren't willing to talk to nurses may be missing out. In many epilepsy centers and neurology practices, doctors have limited time and nurses are extremely knowledgeable and can provide invaluable information and recommendations. How much information is exchanged between doctor to nurse varies by the practice and the specific situation, but you should feel comfortable requesting that the doctor be informed of what you tell the nurse.

Physician Assistants

Physician assistants help doctors obtain the medical history, examine the patient, recommend therapy, draw blood, and order tests. In addition, they can consult with doctors and fulfill many other functions, including (in most states) prescribing medication.

The Social Worker/Counselor

Social workers play an important role on the medical team, yet social workers who have experience in children with epilepsy are often found only in large epilepsy centers. If you can't find one close to your home, ask your doctor or other patients in the area for a reference. The social worker assists in educating the parents about epilepsy and helps parents identify resources such as epilepsy centers, special education programs, home health aides, medical insurance benefits, referral to advocacy groups, and parent networks. The social worker provides counseling and allows parents to discuss personal and social issues that may not be addressed by other members of the team. This counselor may also facilitate further communication between the parent and the child's medical team. Counseling can be beneficial not just for parents, but also for children, helping to answer any questions they may have about their seizures and to facilitate their coping.

The Electroencephalography Technician

An EEG is a recording of the brain's electrical activity (see Chapter 5). It is performed by an EEG technician. The EEG technician will ask you questions about your child's background, apply the leads to your child's head, record the EEG itself, and prepare the results to be reviewed by the physician.

The Pharmacist

Pharmacists fill prescriptions and dispense medication ordered for your child. They're also available to further discuss any potential side effects of a particular medication and the interactions of medications with each other. Pharmacists can also dispense information about over-the-counter, herbal, and other products. You should tell both your physician and your pharmacist about any herbal or natural supplements your child takes regularly. Medication can be expensive; together with your physician, the pharmacist can help you monitor the cost of drugs and the risks and benefits of brand name versus generic drugs. It is wise to check with your doctor before changing from a brand name to a generic formulation.

Parents are sometimes more comfortable speaking to their pharmacist regarding medication treatment than they are with the doctor. Be aware, however, that while pharmacists are very knowledgeable about medications and can provide expert information, they cannot substitute for physicians. To ensure that your child is receiving optimal treatment and the best chance at seizure control, you should speak to the involved medical team regarding any concerns about medications.

Epilepsy Associations, Support Groups, and Online Communities

The Epilepsy Foundation's (EF's) local affiliates and community epilepsy center-based support groups are valuable resources, as are online communities and support groups. These groups are sometimes directed by social workers or counselors. Depending on the specific group, services may include support group meetings to discuss social and related issues, lectures on health issues, referrals for vocational rehabilitation, lectures to school children and school nurses about epilepsy, and assistance with medical and other referrals. Online support groups have been formed around particular epilepsy syndromes and issues. Many such groups and discussion boards find a home on the EF's epilepsy.com website. The EF and many other patient groups and family organizations host active communities on Facebook. Large epilepsy centers often host parent networks, which are a good resource for meeting other families going through similar circumstances. These networks can also connect kids—patients and siblings—with their peers.

SPECIALTY MEMBERS OF THE HEALTH CARE TEAM

Each child's health care team is defined by his specific needs. In epilepsy centers, a consultation with a neuropsychologist and psychiatrist is common, especially when surgery is being considered. In addition, children who have difficulties with academics often benefit from a neuropsychological evaluation to identify disorders such as attention deficit disorder and to assist with school placement. Specialists in physical therapy, occupational therapy, music therapy, speech therapy, and special education can play an important role in the care of selected patients.

The Neuropsychologist

Neuropsychologists assess patients' intellectual and behavioral functions. In the case of a child with epilepsy, a neuropsychologist or an assistant is able to administer tests to help identify relative strengths and weaknesses in areas such as thinking, reasoning, memory, language, perception, motor ability, and behavior. These tests are essential if epilepsy surgery is being considered for the child. Neuropsychologists can also monitor for changes in certain intellectual functions. In addition, an evaluation by a neuropsychologist can assist in academic planning and implementing a plan or individualized education program (IEP) for academic accommodations.

The Psychologist

Psychologists can help children and their families understand and cope with epilepsy. They can guide the family in learning to live more positively and productively. As a parent, you may be overwhelmed by your child's diagnosis. Remember, you need to take care of your own mental health as well as the health of your child. The psychologist's counseling role is similar to that of a social worker: The psychologist can help treat mood disorders and problems with self-esteem and independence that can occur in children and adolescent patients. Psychologists can also be a much-needed resource when it comes to talking out the life stresses that result from epilepsy, the disorder's treatment, and its consequences. Psychologists can provide cognitive behavioral therapy, a form of psychotherapy that focuses on changing thought patterns to change how people feel and act.

The Physical Therapist

Physical therapists help children who have disorders of movement, coordination, or sensation, allowing these children to become more physically able. Developmental milestones, gross motor function, and fine motor function are monitored closely as children grow. When children have delays in these areas, physical therapists use stretching, exercises, and skills development to enhance mobility and coordination.

The Occupational Therapist

Occupational therapists help children with disorders that affect their ability to perform daily tasks, especially tasks requiring fine motor control, such as writing.

The Speech-Language Pathologist

Speech-language pathologists assist children who have speech, language, and swallowing disorders. When a child has difficulty feeding, they can direct the child toward appropriate feeding therapy and oral motor exercises.

The Comprehensive Epilepsy Center

Epilepsy centers are valuable resources for any children who have unresolved problems related to definite or suspected epilepsy. Children may be referred to a comprehensive epilepsy center for a single outpatient visit—for assessment of their current diagnosis and therapy—or for long-term care.

FINANCIAL ISSUES AND INSURANCE COVERAGE

Most doctors and hospitals have office managers, business managers, or other administrative personnel who can address your financial concerns and answer questions about insurance coverage. In cases of financial hardship, many doctors are willing to accept payment plans or reduced fees. Insurances vary in their coverage and access to specialty care, such as care by an epileptologist (an epilepsy specialist). EF affiliates often know of doctors who accept certain insurances/reduced rates and free clinics.

SECOND OPINIONS AND CHANGING DOCTORS

As a parent, you are your child's advocate. You should feel comfortable with your child's medical team and be confident that all aspects of your child's health care are being met. If you don't feel this confidence and believe that your child's doctor is not meeting your child's and family's needs, it may be worth obtaining a second opinion or changing physicians. Before doing this, however, you should consider the areas in which you feel uncertain. In many cases, parents begin to feel more comfortable after asking additional questions of their doctor or raising issues that they're concerned about. If you do decide to seek a second opinion, either ask your child's current pediatric neurologist or epileptologist for another epileptologist or obtain a name from a reliable source. Care should be coordinated, which means that the first neurologist/epileptologist should communicate with and send the patient's records to the epileptologist. The child may continue care with the original doctor, but you should be comfortable switching if you choose.

In some cases, the second doctor may have helpful suggestions regarding tests or changes in therapy. However, often when a second opinion is obtained, the family finds that the first doctor left no stone unturned, and that the second doctor agrees with all aspects of the care recommended by the first physician.

Sometimes it's not a matter of the suggested therapies, but of simple personal chemistry. All relationships depend on personal chemistry, and sometimes the doctor–family mix is just not right. In select cases, communication and trust between parents and the doctor break down. Disagreements can arise, for example, over how much time is spent with the child during the visit, promptness in returning phone calls, finances, antiepileptic drug (AED) side effects, the child's failure to take medication as prescribed, or language difficulties. No matter the reason for making the change, switching doctors can be awkward and uncomfortable. To smooth the transition, be sure to call the original doctor's office and tell the staff that you are changing doctors. The first physician should also be sent a brief note requesting that your child's medical records be forwarded to the new doctor. Don't be shy about asking for this; parents have a legal right to their child's medical records. Call the new doctor's office prior to your first visit to ensure that all the records have arrived. You may incur a charge for copying the records, but there are limits on these charges.

Try to do all you can to avoid burning bridges when changing doctors. In many communities there are only a few neurologists or epileptologists, and you may turn out to like the original one better than the others with whom you consult. Alternatively, the original neurologist may be on call when your child is brought in to the emergency room, and you want to allow for continuity of care.

It may sound as if a daunting number of medical professionals will be involved in your child's care. But you may not encounter all of these experts. Your child's specific syndrome and his individual experience with that syndrome will dictate which experts will be a part of your family's team. Remember, after all, that it is a team. You will be working together to help your child. Sometimes that work involves mainly the pediatric neurologist or epileptologist; at other times, specialists play a large role. Similarly, some children's epilepsies resolve quickly, even without medication; others have a longer road ahead of them.

8 | WHAT'S NEXT? PROGNOSIS FOR CHILDREN WITH EPILEPSY

Once your child has a diagnosis and you have begun meeting members of the medical team, it's time to consider what the future looks like for your child. For the majority of children, that future is seizure-free: Approximately half of children diagnosed with epilepsy no longer have seizures with the first drug and two-thirds after additional therapies. A number of factors can help predict whether your child will fall into this majority group, including:

- The length of time between seizures. The longer the time, the greater the chance for permanent remission, known as *seizure freedom*.

- The age at which she was diagnosed and ease with which her seizures can be controlled. Children who are between 1 and 12 years of age at diagnosis usually have episodes that quickly come under control and have a greater chance of outgrowing seizures.

- Neurological test results. Children with no brain injuries, no abnormalities on the MRI, and normal neurological exams have higher remission rates, unless the cause is genetic, such as a mutation in the SCN1A gene.

On the flip side, children whose seizures take a longer time to come under control have a lower chance of remission. You will usually know if your child's seizures are going to stop with treatment within the first two years of diagnosis. Some seizures, do, however, stop after these two years. As treatments continue to advance, it's becoming more common for children with treatment-resistant epilepsy to later become seizure-free.

An electroencephalogram (EEG) can also be useful in predicting whether a child will outgrow epilepsy, since it can help identify the epilepsy syndrome, and some syndromes are more commonly outgrown. Benign rolandic epilepsy, for example, which has very characteristic EEG spikes, is always outgrown before the patient turns 15 years old. Generalized seizures, diagnosed with a generalized spike-and-wave EEG pattern, are much more likely to be outgrown if the child has the syndrome of generalized absence seizures; in contrast, less than a quarter of patients with juvenile myoclonic epilepsy will have a remission of seizures.

When children stop having seizures for a year or longer—either on or off medication—it is natural to assume that the child is "in the clear" and epilepsy will likely be outgrown. This depends, however, on many factors, the most important of which is the epilepsy syndrome. For children on medication, the second most important factor is regular adherence to taking the medication. When seizures recur after a period of seizure freedom, it is often frustrating. Sometimes the reason for these new seizures is unknown, explained only by the fact that the child continues to have a tendency toward seizures. The 19th-century English neurologist, Sir William Gowers, suggested that "seizures beget seizures"—if the brain has one seizure, it is more likely to have another, because your brain "learns" how to have a seizure. This concept remains unproved, and in children, evidence suggests that treatment has no effect on remission.

GETTING OFF MEDICATIONS: WILL THE SEIZURES RETURN?

Medication is effective at controlling epilepsy in a large number of children, but what happens when the medication is stopped can vary. In about 20 to 30 percent of these children, the seizures will start again once they stop taking the drugs. So, how do you decide (with the help of your child's doctor) that it's time to withdraw medication? Ideally, a child should be seizure-free for two years while on medication before transitioning off medication. An EEG without spikes may further increase the odds of remaining seizure free when off medications. Again, each case is unique and there are exceptions to this general rule. The goal is to control seizures and provide the best chance for long-term seizure freedom. The child's extracurricular activities—such as driving, babysitting, or lifeguarding, if the patient is an adolescent—can influence the decision of when to withdraw medication, too.

The time course of medication withdrawal should be discussed with your doctor. Antiepileptic drugs (AEDs) should never be stopped abruptly unless directed by the medical team. The rate of withdrawal will depend on the epilepsy syndrome, specific AED, total dose, and many other factors.

TREATMENT-RESISTANT EPILEPSY

We've talked about children whose seizures come under control with medication, but approximately 25 percent of children newly diagnosed with epilepsy have symptoms that are not controlled with antiepilepsy drugs. These children have treatment-resistant epilepsy. Risk factors for treatment-resistant epilepsy include having focal epilepsy, more than one seizure type, abnormalities on a neurological examination or imaging studies, long duration of active epilepsy, and failure of initial medications to control seizure. Childhood epilepsy with a genetic abnormality such as tuberous sclerosis, Dravet syndrome, CDKL5, Aicardi syndrome, and Dup 15q are often treatment resistant. In children who are highly suspected of having genetic-based epilepsy, diagnosis can help identify therapies and suggest medications to avoid, as well as provide support through disease organizations formed by parents whose children have the same disorder. For some children who haven't found seizure relief from drugs (often this means that they have tried more than two medications without benefit), dietary therapy should be considered (see Chapter 11).

WHAT HAPPENS TO UNTREATED EPILEPSY?

What happens following the decision to not treat seizures and the natural history of untreated epilepsy are not well known. In some cases, as with benign rolandic epilepsy, the epilepsy remits without treatment. Often this condition does not require medication intervention, but instead benefits from close monitoring and seizure precautions that include good sleep hygiene.

No well-designed studies have answered the question of whether or not treatment, or early treatment, reduces the risk for chronic or treatment-resistant epilepsy. Each child's case and seizure history is individualized and should be considered when discussing treatment.

ASSOCIATED DISORDERS

For some children and adolescents, the disorders that can be associated with epilepsy—such as depression, anxiety, memory loss, and attention deficit hyperactivity disorder—may be more disabling than the seizures. These associated problems (which only affect some epilepsy patients) can result from multiple factors, including underlying brain disorder, recurrent (especially tonic–clonic) seizures and treatment-resistant focal seizures, antiepilepsy drugs, and psychological issues. The medical team can work with the child and family on effective strategies to minimize these problems, often by controlling seizures with the lowest effective dose of medication. Healthy diet, exercise, sleep, and social life are also extremely important for the child's overall health and well-being. Childhood obesity, a growing problem in the general population, can complicate treatment. Some antiepilepsy and psychiatric medications can cause weight gain (or weight loss). Apart from frequent and uncontrolled seizures, it is difficult to predict which patients are at risk of developing cognitive and behavioral complications of epilepsy. If you do notice any cognitive or behavioral changes in your child while she's being treated for epilepsy, be sure to talk to your child's doctor about the changes, so that treatment can be adjusted, if necessary. Notably, many cognitive, behavioral, and physical comorbid disorders associated with epilepsy precede epilepsy.

CAN SEIZURES BE FATAL?

Single seizures are almost never life-threatening. But status epilepticus—seizures that are longer than 10 minutes, or a series of seizures without the child returning to normal awareness in between—is a medical emergency and may, *rarely,* cause permanent injury or death if treatment is delayed or ineffective. Although very rare, status epilepticus is something to be aware of, since quick treatment can make the difference.

You'll also want to avoid situations that can lead to serious accidents and injuries; although these are uncommon, children with epilepsy have higher rates of accidents and drownings. For example, a complex partial seizure may cause a child to ride her bike into oncoming traffic without awareness. Driving a motor vehicle is dangerous for an older adolescent who has episodes of impaired consciousness. Water can provide an added hazard, and death from drowning is more common among people with epilepsy (and can even occur in the bathtub). Children and adolescents should never swim alone, and special attention must be paid in lakes and oceans, where currents and limited visibility in the water can prevent rescue.

In working to protect your child from injuries, you'll want to strike a balance between safety and allowing your child to lead an active, productive, enjoyable life. It is important that you evaluate the risks as your child chooses and takes part in various activities, but also that you continue to allow her to keep up with her peers. Most injuries occur during normal daily activities—and you can't bubble-wrap your child. Even children with poorly controlled epilepsy can participate in most activities with some precautions. Children without epilepsy suffer injuries frequently.

You should be aware of sudden unexpected death in epilepsy (SUDEP)—a leading cause of death among people with epilepsy—but you can take comfort in knowing that SUDEP is rare among children. In pediatric epilepsy, SUDEP is occasionally seen in adolescents with ongoing tonic–clonic seizures—whether because seizures cannot be controlled with medication, or because the adolescent forgets to take her medications or engages in behaviors that increase the risk of seizures (for example, by drinking alcohol or going without enough sleep). Yet SUDEP very rarely takes the life of a young child who has infrequent seizures. Most SUDEPs occur in sleep, and the child is found face down. SUDEP's cause is not fully understood, but some combination of the brain shutting down after a tonic–clonic seizure and breathing difficulties is considered a major factor; in some cases, heart-rhythm problems likely contribute. The only prevention for SUDEP is controlling seizures. Several studies suggest that SUDEP is less common when epilepsy patients are monitored during sleep. Unfortunately, no studies have assessed the potential benefits of seizure alarms, monitoring, special pillows, or seizure alert dogs in preventing SUDEP. Many parents use sound monitors or seizure detection devices to alarm them when their child has a seizure (see http://www.dannydid.org/epilepsy-sudep/

devices-technology/). Since there is no evidence that these monitors prevent SUDEP, lack of availability should not be a reason to deny children sleepovers or summer camps. Antisuffocation pillows are also an option, as are seizure alert dogs who can help parents identify nocturnal and also daytime seizures.

Remember, SUDEP is rare in pediatric epilepsy. In some groups of children—for example, those with childhood absence epilepsy—SUDEP has never been documented. In children with recurrent tonic–clonic seizures, however, new therapies to control seizures, including diet and surgery, should be considered, as well as safety measures to help monitor seizures. More information can be found at epilepsy.com/sudep-institute.

YOUR CHILD'S LONG-TERM OUTLOOK

Many children with epilepsy lead normal lives and have few or no restrictions on their social or physical activities. For other children, side effects of medication and ongoing seizures can cause difficulties, and their daily lives may be impacted by additional medical, neurological, and psychiatric problems. Where your child falls on this spectrum depends greatly on the types of seizures your child experiences and the syndrome she has, as well as the treatment chosen. When considering drug therapy, surgery, or dietary modifications, you'll want to aim not simply at reducing seizures, but at giving your child the fullest, most enjoyable life possible.

The emotional and medical problems that tend to occur alongside epilepsy are often underappreciated, and addressing them can be as important to your child's health and quality of life as controlling seizures. In many cases, the impact of the other disorders is far greater than the effect of epilepsy. Intensive attention to these problems is extremely important.

9 | PRINCIPLES OF DRUG THERAPY FOR EPILEPSY

In choosing a treatment for your child, the goal is to eliminate seizures, minimize side effects, and allow for a happy childhood filled with rich social, recreational, and educational experiences. Sometimes this goal is reached with no treatment at all. In children with infrequent or mild seizures, for example, daily medication may not be needed and only a "rescue" drug will be prescribed (for use solely if a seizure is prolonged). But for most children with recurrent seizures, medication is recommended and the use of this medication outweighs any risks and side effects. Which particular drug will be prescribed depends on the type of epilepsy (e.g., focal versus generalized), the epilepsy syndrome, and any other conditions the child may have. In general, antiepileptic drugs (AEDs) are most effective for severe seizures (tonic–clonic seizures), intermediate in effectiveness for moderate-intensity seizures (complex partial seizures), and least effective in fully controlling mild seizures (simple partial seizures). For children with generalized epilepsies, tonic–clonic seizures are more completely controlled with AEDs than myoclonic or absence seizures. In addition to choosing a drug, your medical team will have to determine how large a dose should be given and what's next if the medication doesn't work or isn't tolerated.

There is rarely one best drug for a child. In most cases, any of several antiepileptic medications will prove similarly effective, giving your medical team a number of options. The difference is in each drug's side effects. You, your child (if old enough), and the doctor should discuss the pros and cons of each drug, paying special attention to the frequency of dosing (the fewer times of day the better; the sooner your child learns to swallow pills the better, as extended-release preparations can minimize frequency of dosing and side effects), side effects (such as tiredness, weight gain, or loss), and cost. Chapter 10 reviews individual AEDs. Here we talk about them as an overall class of drugs.

Although AEDs control seizures in most children, they do not *cure* epilepsy. This is why people often remark, "These drugs don't really treat the epilepsy, they just control seizures. They are like Band-Aids." There is truth in that statement. If a genetic disorder, scar tissue, or an abnormal group of blood vessels in the brain causes seizures, AEDs will not repair these problems. These medications suppress seizures but do not fix the underlying cause. Being on medications for one, two, four, or five years is associated with the same rate of remission when AEDs are stopped. That is, if a child is on an AED and is seizure free, the chance that seizures will recur if medications are stopped are the same if the child is on medication for one year or five years.

GOALS OF DRUG THERAPY

The goals of treatment, whether drug-based or not, are simple: no seizures, no side effects, good quality of life. For some children this is easily attained, but for others, the balance between seizure control/side effects and a full life is challenging, making compromises unavoidable. As with all aspects in epilepsy treatment, finding this balance relies on clear communication between doctor and parent. If your child goes on AEDs, you and your child's doctor should openly discuss what to expect from the medication, what is tolerable in terms of side effects, what your child is experiencing while on the drug(s), and the overall impact that seizures and any of the drug's side effects are having on the child's quality of life. Older children and adolescents must be involved in this dialogue as well.

Troublesome side effects should never be accepted without attempts to reduce or eliminate them. Some parents fear that if they complain about a medication, the doctor will reduce the dosage and a seizure will occur; other parents believe that side effects are a necessary evil (sometimes they are, but not always). Some doctors incorrectly label complaints of side effects as psychological or attribute them to other factors, especially if the child is on a low dose or if the doctor is not familiar with the particular side effect. Some children are extremely sensitive to medications and do experience problems on low dosages. In other cases, however, doctors mislabel in the opposite direction: blaming medications for minor problems that the drugs did not contribute to. In addition, with children who take medications over many years, it can be hard to separate a side effect from "who they are." The best way to sort out these issues is by carefully observing the potential side effects: How soon did they begin after initiation or increase in a medication? Do they often occur at a similar time after a drug is taken? How long do they last? What makes them better?

How AEDs Work AEDs help restore balance to the brain's chemical and electrical activity. To put it simply, seizures result where there's too much excitation (electrical activity) or too little inhibition (quieting of the electrical activity) in a person's brain. AEDs work in a variety of ways to either reduce the excess excitation or increase the lowered inhibition. For example, many AEDs influence the ion channels that regulate how much of an electrically charged ion (e.g., sodium, calcium, or potassium) enters a nerve cell. Others alter the activity of neurotransmitters and their receptors, such as gamma-amino butyric acid

(GABA), the brain's main inhibitory neurotransmitter. (See Table 9.1 for more information about how specific drugs work.)

Once a drug is chosen, your doctor will have to determine the correct dose, by which we mean: the least amount of medication that will protect your child against seizures, even during periods of stress and sleep deprivation (which are impossible to fully avoid!) or the occasional missed dose. A dose that's less than this may result in breakthrough seizures, while a larger dose can result in side effects. The "right" dose depends on individual factors such as absorption and metabolism of medication, severity of epilepsy, and lifestyle.

How Long Does It Take for an AED to Start Working? The time between when your child takes his first dose of an antiepilepsy medication and when that medication starts to take effect has to do with a number of factors, including the way and rate at which that particular drug is absorbed by the body and how long it takes that drug to reach its peak effect. As for how long the effect of the drug lasts, that depends on factors such as the drug's half-life and steady state, all explained in this chapter.

TABLE 9.1: MECHANISMS OF ANTIEPILEPTIC DRUG ACTION

Decrease Excitation (Reduce the Excessive Electrical Activity)

Decrease Flow in Sodium Channels

carbamazepine, **eslicarbazepine**, felbamate, **lacosamide**, **lamotrigine**, **oxcarbazepine**, phenobarbital, **phenytoin**, rufinamide, topiramate, zonisamide

Decrease Flow in Calcium Channels

ethosuximide, felbamate, gabapentin, levetiracetam, pregabalin, zonisamide

Decrease Flow in Potassium Channels

retigabine

Decrease Action of Excitatory Neurotransmitter Glutamate

felbamate, lamotrigine, **perampanel**, topiramate

Increase Inhibition

Increase Action of Brain's Inhibitory Neurotransmitter GABA

benzodiazepines, gabapentin, **phenobarbital**, **tiagabine**, topiramate, valproate, **vigabatrin**

Bind to a Specific Protein and Alter Synaptic Vesicles

levetiracetam

Bolded text indicates that this category is considered a primary mechanism of action for the drug.

Absorption

Oral medication passes through the stomach and is absorbed in the small intestine. From there, many drugs are metabolized (broken down) in the liver and then enter into the bloodstream. Other drugs are eliminated by the kidneys in an unchanged (not metabolized) form. Eventually, AEDs reach the brain.

Peak Effect

When a drug is at its "peak effect," it is at its maximum concentration in your child's bloodstream and is having the maximum impact in treating your child's seizures. How long it takes for a drug to reach this peak varies. An oral dose of medication will reach its peak, or maximum, blood level a minimum of 30 minutes and a maximum of six hours after it has been administered, depending on the specific drug, its form (liquid, tablet, capsule, slow-release form), and, in some cases, the food consumed before taking it. In general, absorption—and thus the time to peak effect—is faster for liquids, intermediate for immediate-release capsules and tablets, and slowest for "long-acting" or "extended-release" preparations. The properties of selected AEDs when used as sole therapy are summarized in Table 10.1.

Half-Life

The goal with AEDs is to maintain a relatively constant level of the drug in the blood, ensuring a steady level of seizure control. A drug's half-life is the time required for the drug's peak concentration in the blood to drop by 50 percent (Figure 9.1). In the same way that some drugs take effect faster than others, some lose that effect faster. Drugs with longer half-lives keep blood levels (and thus seizure control) more stable and can be taken less frequently. Drugs with short half-lives often have to be taken several times a day to keep the levels stable. If the blood level isn't stable—if there are swings between periods of high levels of the drug and then low levels—there's a risk of adverse side effects during periods of high blood levels alternating with seizures during periods of low levels. In select patients, however, drugs with short half-lives can be taken less frequently, because the effect on the brain is long-lasting. Overall, half-lives are shorter in younger children and progressively increase as the child ages. Genetic factors also influence how an individual child metabolizes a medication.

Some drugs such as carbamazepine, gabapentin, levetiracetam, pregabalin, and tiagabine have a relatively short half-life (less than 10 hours); some, such as clobazam, eslicarbazepine, lamotrigine, topiramate, and phenytoin, have an intermediate half-life (approximately 18–24 hours); and some, such as phenobarbital, zonisamide, and the major metabolite of clobazam, have a long half-life

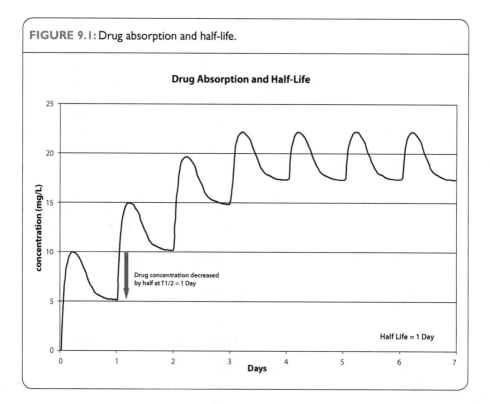

FIGURE 9.1: Drug absorption and half-life.

(more than 40 hours). (See Chapter 10 for details on specific drugs.) Different preparations of the same drugs often have different half-lives and reach peak level at different times. For example, carbamazepine is available as a tablet for swallowing, a chewable tablet, a sustained-release tablet for swallowing, and an elixir. Each form has a different half-life. Because of these differences, switching to a rapidly absorbed or shorter half-life form of the same drug can cause a higher peak level, bringing on more side effects, and/or lower end-of-dose levels, creating greater seizure risk. When drugs are used in combination, the half-life of each drug may change as well.

Elixirs are usually more rapidly absorbed and have shorter half-lives. Sustained-release products and gradual release forms have longer half-lives and produce steadier drug blood levels, meaning that doses can be taken less often without wide swings in the blood levels. Still, children whose seizures only occur around sleep times may do best with an immediate-release form of a medication (with an intermediate half-life) taken only once daily before bedtime. In such cases, the medication's effects are focused on the times when seizures are most likely to occur, and potential daytime side effects are minimized.

Steady State

Steady state (or equilibrium) is what we call the situation where the level of the drug in the blood (*drug blood level*) is fairly constant when the patient is on a specific dosage. In other words, steady state is when the amount of drug taken and the amount being metabolized and excreted are equal. In most cases, steady state is the goal—giving a child maximum seizure control without spikes in side effects. It takes approximately five times longer to reach equilibrium on a drug than the drug's half-life.

Even at equilibrium, drug levels fluctuate over the course of the day and from day to day. Depending on the rate of absorption and other factors that influence this rate (for example, taking some drugs after meals slows absorption), there will be peaks in the drug blood level within hours after the drug is taken, and also troughs (low points) just before a new dose is taken, especially if there is a long interval between doses. Drugs with short half-lives lead to more of this type of fluctuation, though taking these drugs more frequently can reduce this fluctuation. Dose-related side effects are most common at peak levels and a seizure is more likely to occur during times of trough levels. Blood levels can also be influenced by other medications being taken concurrently, viral infections, menstrual cycles, genetics, and other factors. Even taking all of these factors into consideration, blood levels are not completely stable. If your child has a trough drug level of 60 when taking 500 mg of valproic acid, the level could be 5 to 25 percent higher or lower when the level is repeated at the same time of day a few weeks later.

SIDE EFFECTS OF AEDS

The side effects associated with AEDs can be minor or severe. They can be short-lasting and reversible, or long-lasting and, very rarely, irreversible (see Table 10.2). Most, luckily, are mild and transient. Before starting a medication, you (and your child, if old enough to understand) should know what to expect. Some fatigue, abdominal discomfort, or dizziness is common during the first weeks of taking an AED, but if the medication is started at a low dosage and increased slowly, and if the patient is aware of what to expect, these effects are usually tolerable. They tend to stop after several weeks or months, as tolerance develops. If intolerable side effects occur even with low doses, the drug should be discontinued (after discussion with the doctor) and another drug should be tried. Loss of bone density can be a progressive problem related to some AEDs and is more common than generally appreciated by doctors and patients. If your child is taking any drugs that activate certain liver enzymes—carbamazepine, phenobarbital, phenytoin, primidone, topiramate, and valproate are among these drugs—you should talk to your child's doctor about whether he should take calcium and vitamin D supplements, and you should also talk about obtaining bone density measurements.

Side effects related to AEDs are broadly divided into two types: those that are unpredictable and not related to dosage or blood level (*idiosyncratic*), and those that are related to the dose and to blood level (*dose-related*).

Side Effects That Aren't Related to the Drug's Dosage

Idiosyncratic side effects are typically due to an allergic (immunological) reaction to the drug. These side effects include rash, fever, inflammation of the liver or pancreas, and a serious reduction in the number of white blood cells (which fight infection), platelets (control bleeding), and red blood cells (carry oxygen; see Table 10.2). Dangerous but very rare idiosyncratic reactions such as aplastic anemia (bone marrow failure) and liver failure usually occur within a few weeks or months of beginning a drug. Other idiosyncratic side effects include hair loss, swollen lymph glands, and mouth ulcers.

Life-threatening problems related to AEDs are extremely rare. Fewer than one person in 75,000 who take AEDs will die as a result; the average American has a 10-fold higher chance of dying in a motor vehicle accident every year. The more serious risks of AEDs include rashes that cause a peeling of the skin or involve mucous membranes (like those in the mouth), infection that results from a low white blood cell count, serious bleeding as the result of a low platelet count, liver damage, or pancreas damage. Other risks include kidney stones, significant weight gain or loss, gum overgrowth, a drop in blood sodium, and neuropathy.

When To Call a Doctor

Doctors should be notified immediately if a child develops excessive bleeding, severe abdominal pain, fever, unusual infections, or other unusual symptoms while taking an AED.

If a rash or fever develops after a new medication is prescribed, call the doctor immediately. Rashes usually begin 5 to 18 days after a medication is started and usually the earliest areas to be affected are the chest, back, and parts of the extremities near the trunk. If the rash is an allergic reaction, it may be preceded by fever and/or swollen glands several days earlier. Many rashes are mild and result from causes other than the drug—such as viruses, bacteria, allergic reactions unrelated to medication, laundry detergent, insect bites, and so on—so the doctor's first task is to decide if the rash is a side effect or if it stems from another cause. In patients taking more than one drug, the most recently started drug has probably caused the rash (if the rash is a side effect). A drug-related rash usually resolves shortly after the medication is discontinued. The child should be seen in person by a doctor if the rash is severe, and in some cases steroids may be prescribed. Diphenhydramine (Benadryl) should be used sparingly, as it may slightly increase the likelihood of seizures. Appendix C reviews over-the-counter drugs that can lower the seizure threshold; see also Table 9.2.

TABLE 9.2: ANTIEPILEPTIC DRUGS THAT MAY AGGRAVATE SEIZURES

Drug	Seizure Type Affected
Carbamazepine	Absence, myoclonic, JME, LGS, Dravet
Eslicarbazepine	Absence, myoclonic, JME, LGS, Dravet
Ethosuximide	Myoclonic, tonic–clonic
Gabapentin	Absence, myoclonic, LGS
Lamotrigine	Myoclonic, atonic, JME, LGS, Dravet
Oxcarbazepine	Absence, myoclonic, JME, LGS, Dravet
Phenytoin	Absence, myoclonic, JME, LGS, Dravet
Pregabalin	Absence, myoclonic, LGS
Tiagabine	Absence
Vigabatrin	Absence, myoclonic, LGS

Over-the-counter drugs that can worsen seizure control are listed in Appendix C.

JME, juvenile myoclonic epilepsy; LGS, Lennox–Gastaut Syndrome.

Side Effects Directly Related to AED Dosage

Dose-related side effects are more common than idiosyncratic side effects, and can often be managed by decreasing the dose temporarily until the patient becomes more "used to the drug" (that is, until tolerance develops). In other cases, giving small doses more frequently, giving the medication after meals, or giving a larger dose at bedtime may reduce or eliminate adverse effects. The one type of dose-related effect that can't be managed in these ways is an allergic reaction. If you child has an allergic reaction to a drug, that drug will usually need to be discontinued and a new drug tried in its place.

When the dosage of a drug is increased, the drug blood level may become too high for the child to tolerate and troublesome effects, called *toxicity*, will occur. It is difficult to predict the exact dosage or blood level of a drug that will cause toxicity in a given person. The recommended dosage of a drug, known as its "therapeutic range," is typically one in which most children have good seizure control and mild or no side effects. However, there is great variability between children in what dose is tolerated. Some children do best on a drug when it is slightly out of the therapeutic range, and experts often don't agree on the specific therapeutic range for specific drugs.

Metabolites (substances that are products of a drug's metabolism) may contribute to toxicity. Many metabolites are *inactive*, but some drugs used to treat seizures (such as carbamazepine, clobazam, and valproate) produce *active* metabolites—substances derived from the liver's "digestion"—that can have antiepileptic effects and also side effects of their own. Measuring only blood levels in patents using carbamazepine, clobazam or valproate may be misleading, as the metabolites may contribute to any problem that arises. Other drugs can also alter the level of active metabolites.

Dose-related side effects almost never cause dangerous or permanent problems and typically resolve with lower doses. Spreading the dose more evenly or frequently throughout the day, having the child take medications with meals or at bedtime, and lowering the dose can often help dose-related side effects. These side effects are more likely when two or more drugs are used (when more than one drug is used, it's called *polytherapy*) and when blood levels exceed the therapeutic range; however, some sensitive patients experience problems on a single drug even when the blood level is in the therapeutic range. Reducing the number of drugs or dosage can reduce side effects.

An important challenge is distinguishing other common problems that are unrelated to the medications such as tension and migraine headaches, stomach viruses, near-sightedness, as well as comorbid problems such as attention deficit disorder. If you are concerned about side effects, you should discuss them with the doctor or other members of the health care team.

Dose-related side effects (toxicity) tend to fall into one of three categories: bodily and general neurological effects, cognitive effects, and behavioral effects.

Bodily and General Neurological Effects

Common dose-related side effects are dizziness, tiredness, stomach discomfort, increased or decreased appetite, headache, tremor, unsteadiness, and blurred or double vision. These are the most frequent side effects of antiepileptic drugs. At higher or toxic dosage, more severe forms of all these problems can occur: vomiting, falling, or marked weight gain or loss (see Table 10.2).

Cognitive Effects

AEDs often reduce seizures by reducing the excitability of brain cells. They can also dampen normal brain activity and impair cognitive function, hampering a child's attention and concentration, memory, mood, drive to do things, and speed of mental thought and movement. Benzodiazepines, phenobarbital, primidone, and topiramate are among the drugs associated with increased rates of cognitive problems.

Behavioral Effects

AEDs can cause anxiety, irritability, or depression, and on rare occasions they cause mania (abnormally elevated mood, energy, and activity), paranoia, or psychosis. Although AED-related behavioral problems are usually mild and transient, they can occasionally be severe and chronic. It is difficult to predict who will develop behavioral side effects. Children with prior behavioral and developmental disorders may be more susceptible, and behavioral problems are more common when a drug dose is rapidly increased, when high doses are used, and when multiple AEDs (polytherapy) are used. The drugs ACTH, clobazam, clonazepam, levetiracetam, phenobarbital, mysoline, rufinamide, topiramate, vigabatrin, and zonisamide are most commonly associated with increased rates of behavioral problems.

TOLERANCE

Tolerance refers to the decreased effect of a drug or class of drugs as the result of a medication's repeated administration. With tolerance, the drug becomes less potent over time and larger doses must be used to obtain the same effect, whether the effect is good (seizure control) or bad (sleepiness). There are two main forms of tolerance. *Metabolic tolerance* is when a person's body becomes more effective at eliminating the drug; for example, the liver metabolizes it more rapidly. *Pharmacodynamic tolerance* is when there's an adaptive change in the tissue or organ affected by the drug. For example, long-term use of benzodiaze-pines reduces the sensitivity of a person's GABA receptors, so a given dose of the drug becomes less effective. Regularly using one drug of this type (for example, clonazepam taken by mouth) will produce tolerance to another type (such as rectal diazepam or intranasal midazolam).

A very small amount of tolerance can occur when taking most AEDs, but this minor level of tolerance usually does not affect seizure control. Occasionally, a child does well with a new drug for several weeks or months, but over time the drug becomes less effective and seizures recur or become more frequent (the "honeymoon effect").

Benzodiazepines are the AEDs most often associated with tolerance affecting the therapeutic benefits. These drugs are among the most powerful in the emer-gency control of serious and prolonged seizures, but because of the tolerance issue are less effective in long-term treatment. The relative exception to this rule appears to be clobazam, which does have good long-term effectiveness.

MISSED DOSES

One day we received a panicked call from a parent whose child had his first tonic–clonic in several years. "How could this have happened?" "Let's start with the common factors—any missed medications, sleep deprivation, gastrointestinal (GI) illness…?""Well, he missed his dose last night, but that could not have caused the seizures.""Why not?""Because he often misses a dose." Because your child gets away with a missed dose multiple times, don't be surprised when a large seizure occurs. Seizure occurrence is a complex issue—essentially a probabilistic event for which we understand many but by no means all of the factors that are involved. The more intense and prolonged a single factor (say, multiple missed dosages in a row versus a single missed dose), the more likely it is that a seizure will occur. Provocative factors are synergistic: combining them can exponentially increase the likelihood of seizure occurrence. The leading cause of seizures in someone who is well controlled is missed medication.

Parents, older children, and adolescents sometimes forget to give or take a dose. Perhaps they've overslept and, in the rush to get to work or school, forgot the morning medication. Or perhaps a child has simply fallen asleep before taking the bedtime dose. Given the differences in epilepsy type, seizure control between patients, and the variations in drug half-lives and other factors, there's no hard-and-fast rule about what to do when a dose is missed. Instead, ask your doctor what to do if this happens. As a general rule, if a single dose is missed, we recommend that it be taken as soon as possible. Avoid "doubling up" when it's time for the next dose, as this may lead to side effects; instead, take the missed dose as soon as possible and then take the next scheduled dose after an interval of at least two hours, often with some food to delay absorption of the second dose. If your child misses two doses within the same 24-hour period, it is usually recommended that one dose be taken as soon as it is remembered and the second missed dose two to four hours later. If your child misses more than two doses of medication in one 24-hour period, or if he doesn't take his medication entirely for more than 24 hours, call your doctor's office.

Again, it's best to consult with your doctor ahead of time to have a plan if a dose is missed, since the best course of action—or inaction—depends greatly on the child and the epilepsy, the medication missed and its dosage, and other medications that the child takes.

IS THE DOSE AFFECTED WHEN YOUR CHILD IS SICK?

Vomiting and diarrhea both impair absorption. This fact can't be emphasized enough. Vomiting and diarrhea can reduce the absorption of medication, lowering blood levels, and possibly causing seizures—especially in children with illnesses that already physically and emotionally stress them.

The interval between oral intake and absorption of a medication varies. When GI function is abnormal, as occurs with a GI virus or food poisoning—two common causes of vomiting and diarrhea—absorption can be delayed and reduced. Although most tablets are usually absorbed within an hour or two, a GI illness can delay this considerably (pill fragments in vomit are one way to tell that the medicine was not fully absorbed). Repeating the dose can sometimes fix the problem, but often not in the case of longer illness, as absorption will remain disrupted. In these cases, a dissolvable clonazepam wafer on the tongue may be a short-term solution.

If an illness is prolonged, or if your child has watery diarrhea for more than four to six hours (which can lower blood levels), you should notify your physician and consider a temporary increase in dosage or other strategy to help prevent a seizure.

Traveling and Time Zone Changes

Avoid scheduling flights that guarantee sleep deprivation—even in the same time zone! If your daughter normally sleeps until 7:00 a.m., a flight that leaves at 8:00 a.m. may require you to wake her up at 5:30 a.m. to travel to the airport and clear security. Better to schedule a flight that minimizes sleep deprivation.

Traveling across time zones poses three risks for breakthrough seizures: change in the child's sleep–wake (circadian) cycle, sleep deprivation, and reduction in AED levels due to changing schedules. Changing time zones can be a physical and mental stress. Shifting time zones can disrupt sleep. Children with epilepsy should get plenty of sleep for the first one or two days after a greater than one-hour shift in time zone. So if a child travels from New York to Paris, the first few days in Paris and the first few days after returning to New York, he should take it easy and get plenty of sleep.

When traveling across time zones, the amount of medication taken over a 24- or 48-hour period should remain constant or increase slightly, and the interval between doses should be the same or shorter. Because changes in time zones increase the likelihood of sleep deprivation and disrupt the body's clock, better to err on the side of taking slightly too much medication or too-frequent doses than too little.

Each drug has a half-life, the time required for the drug's blood concentration to decline to half of its maximum value. Medications with a short half-life, such as gabapentin, pose a greater problem than those with a longer half-life, such as lamotrigine or zonisamide. For drugs with a short half-life, the interval between doses should be maintained as much as possible. Otherwise, side effects from high drug levels or seizures from low drug levels could result. It's not necessary to use an alarm clock to take the medications at exactly the same interval, however. The timing with long half-life medications is less critical because the drug levels fluctuate less.

If the seizures have been difficult to control, if there are problems with dose-related side effects, or if time-zone differences are confusing, the patient should ask the doctor about taking medications during travel. In some persons, benzodiazepines such as clonazepam may increase sleep time on the plane, decrease jet lag, and reduce the risk of a seizure while traveling. Melatonin can be used to help re-establish a normal sleep pattern.

DRUG ABSORPTION AND FOOD

It's fine to take any AED around mealtime. A full stomach may delay but does not reduce absorption. Side effects due to peak levels, such as blurred vision or dizziness, may be reduced by taking the medicine during or after meals to slow absorption. Peak side effects are most common 30 minutes to several hours after a dose.

FINDING THE RIGHT DRUG

For each type of seizure, one or more AED may be considered the "best" treatment based on its effectiveness and mild side-effect profile (these are called "primary drugs"). If your child is starting drug therapy, one of these primary drugs will probably be recommended first, for his main type of seizure (Table 9.3). Because some medications work well for certain seizure types but are ineffective or even worsen other types, correct seizure diagnosis is essential. And just because the drug chosen has been effective in other patients with your child's seizure type, that doesn't mean it will necessarily be the right fit for your child and his epilepsy. *One child's troublesome drug can be another's miracle.* These medication recommendations are based on studies of the collective experiences of many patients, but there is considerable variation when it comes to people's individual reactions to the drug, in terms of the drugs' effectiveness and side effects. So what works for the majority may not end up being the best course for your child.

TABLE 9.3: PRIMARY AND SECONDARY ANTIEPILEPTIC DRUGS FOR DIFFERENT SEIZURE TYPES AND EPILEPSY SYNDROMES

Seizure Type	Primary Drug	Secondary Drug
Idiopathic (Primary) Generalized		
Absence	Ethosuximide Lamotrigine Valproate	Topiramate Zonisamide
Myoclonic	Levetiracetam Valproate	Clobazam or clonazepam Lamotrigine Topiramate Zonisamide
Tonic–clonic	Lamotrigine Levetiracetam Valproate	Carbamazepine Clobazam Eslicarbazepine Oxcarbazepine Phenytoin Topiramate Zonisamide

(continued)

TABLE 9.3: PRIMARY AND SECONDARY ANTIEPILEPTIC DRUGS FOR DIFFERENT SEIZURE TYPES AND EPILEPSY SYNDROMES (*CONTINUED*)

Seizure Type	Primary Drug	Secondary Drug
Juvenile myoclonic epilepsy syndrome	Lamotrigine Levetiracetam Topiramate Valproate	Acetazolamide Clobazam Clonazepam Primidone
Infantile spasms (West syndrome)	Adrenocorticotropic hormone (ACTH) Vigabatrin	Topiramate Valproate
Lennox–Gastaut syndrome	Lamotrigine Topiramate Valproate	Carbamazepine Clobazam Felbamate Rufinamide Zonisamide
Focal		
Simple partial, complex partial, and secondary generalized tonic–clonic seizures	Carbamazepine Lamotrigine Levetiracetam Oxcarbazepine Zonisamide	Clobazam Eslicarbazepine Gabapentin Perampanel Phenytoin Pregabalin Topiramate Valproate
Benign rolandic epilepsy	Carbamazepine Lamotrigine Oxcarbazepine	Eslicarbazepine Gabapentin Levetiracetam Pregabalin Topiramate Valproate Zonisamide

After your doctor prescribes an AED—doctors will usually start by prescribing just one drug, in hopes that it will be a good fit—your medical team will closely monitor the medication's progress, beginning with a low dose and increasing it slowly (unless your child's condition requires a more rapid build-up). The correct dosage will be when your child's seizures are brought under control with the minimum of side effects. If the drug doesn't seem to be having any impact on your child, a blood test to measure how much drug is in the bloodstream can help determine if he is not receiving the AED (for example, a teenager who frequently forgets), if the drug is being metabolized or eliminated at an unusually rapid rate, or if levels suggest that the drug is being given at too low or high a dose.

In prescribing a drug for your child's main type of seizures, the doctor will also have to consider any other types of seizures the child has experienced, as it's not unusual for epilepsy patients to have several types of seizures. A patient with juvenile myoclonic epilepsy may have myoclonic and tonic–clonic seizures, for example—and while lamotrigine may be effective in controlling tonic–clonic seizures, it may have little effect on, or even increase the frequency of, the myoclonic seizures. In such cases, the benefits of lamotrigine may be outweighed by the costs, and it may be preferable to find a medication that controls all seizure types. In other cases, lamotrigine may be very effective for both seizure types.

Children who can swallow pills often find it easiest to take one small pill once a day, and this can also influence the choice of drug. That's because in some cases, 100 mg of drug A has the same beneficial effect as 10 mg (a much smaller pill) of drug B. Your first goal in selecting medication should always be seizure control with minimal or no side effects, but if these factors are the same with both of these drugs, the change to smaller pills can make taking medication much less of a hassle for your child.

In most patients, there's a single primary AED that will provide the best balance between seizure control and side effects. Some doctors put patients on three or more AEDs at moderate doses instead, but this can increase the chance of side effects and breakthrough seizures. As a result, we highly recommend trying to stick with one drug. If seizures persist while your child is taking a single AED, and this AED causes no side effects, it is usually best to increase the dose until the seizures are controlled or side effects develop rather than adding another medication. The key is to make sure that the increase in dosage is gradual, because rapid dose increases can cause disabling side effects (fatigue, impaired concentration, dizziness) that are considered intolerable. These side effects can cause a potentially effective and well-tolerated medication to be incorrectly dismissed as "intolerable."

This is the route that works in most patients, but not all. If no single drug proves effective in controlling seizures, some patients do end up requiring two, three, or four medications to gain full seizure control. In these cases, the benefits should outweigh the risks. Once a second drug is added, parents and the doctor should track the change in seizure frequency and severity, as well as side effects, with different dosages. Do the benefits of the second drug outweigh any additional side effects and financial cost? For example, a 20 percent reduction in seizure frequency may not be worth the cost of severe tiredness and dizziness. Medication selection and dosage adjustment require open communication between the child, parent, and doctor. Switching to a new AED typically means adding the new one before eliminating the first one, because the child's seizures have to be controlled, as best as possible, during the transition. Once the child is on a therapeutic dose or level of the new medication, the original AED can slowly be tapered and eliminated.

Any changes in medication should be done systematically and be limited to one drug at a time whenever possible. This strategy helps establish a relationship between a change and an effect such as improved seizure control or worsening side effects. If a drug is suspected of causing a side effect, the dose may be gradually reduced and the child observed to see if the side effects diminish or resolve. Even here, coincidence or bias may be the explanation. Confirmation bias is a common human trait that selectively favors information that supports one's beliefs; it afflicts doctors, parents, and patients.

No matter which or how many drugs are involved, you should work with your child's doctor to create a medication schedule that's adapted to your child's lifestyle. The schedule should be one that's convenient, minimizes adverse effects, and controls seizures. Whatever schedule is set, you should never experiment with varying this schedule without discussing these changes with a doctor or nurse first. (Some medications aren't easy to adjust in terms of schedule. For example, drugs like gabapentin have short half-lives and almost always have to be taken more than once a day to be effective in controlling seizures and to minimize side effects. An exception is in children with nocturnal seizures, where a single dose before bedtime can be effective and help reduce or eliminate daytime side effects.)

Secondary AEDs Sometimes the primary drug your child has been prescribed has to be stopped. Perhaps your child has developed a rash or other allergic reaction while on the drug, or has come down with disabling fatigue or another side effect. In these cases, another primary drug is usually tried alone, repeating the fashion in which the first was introduced. Sometimes the primary drug is tolerated without side effects and blood levels are in the high therapeutic range, but it isn't managing to bring the seizures under control. In this case, some experts will try another primary drug or a *secondary* drug (one that is not often the remedy of choice for the situation in question) alone, while others will add another drug to the current regimen (see Table 9.3) without stopping the first. The decision should be based on the potential benefits and side effects of one versus two drugs.

When one medication is added to another medication, it is referred to as *adjunctive therapy*. Use of one medicine is *monotherapy*. The concurrent use of two or more drugs is *polytherapy*. Although some drugs are considered secondary because they tend to have fewer good effects and more bad effects than the drugs categorized as primary, secondary drugs can be very safe and effective. Many epilepsy patients are successfully treated using only secondary drugs. We can't say this enough: Every case of epilepsy is different, as is every child's experience with it. This is why determining a drug treatment plan often isn't a perfect science, but can involve trial and error.

WHAT IF THE DRUG FAILS?

The first attempt at AED therapy may be ineffective for several reasons:

- The child does not have epilepsy.
- The drug is the wrong AED for the child's seizure type or epilepsy syndrome.
- The child didn't take the medication as prescribed.
- The prescribed doses weren't correct for controlling the seizures.
- The child had an allergic reaction (such as rash or hives) to the medication.
- The child experienced medication side effects such as tiredness or nausea.

Could the failure be because the seizure type or epilepsy syndrome has been diagnosed incorrectly? Yes! This kind of misdiagnosis happens to all doctors—from pediatricians to pediatric neurologists and pediatric epilepsy experts—often because they've misinterpreted the patient's clinical history or electroencephalography (EEG), and sometimes because they've relied too heavily on the accepted dogma and bias. Whatever the reason for misdiagnosis, it can lead to the prescription of a drug that isn't right for that particular child's epilepsy.

Another common reason for drug failure is missed doses, which can cause a breakthrough seizure in a patient whose episodes were previously controlled.

Sometimes even when the dose and drug are right, the medication may still fail if it's not scheduled correctly and, as a result, low levels occur at the time when seizures are most likely. For patients whose seizures happen at random times, therapeutic levels of medication should be maintained continuously. For people prone to seizures at specific times of the day or night, doses can be timed to maximize seizure control at these times and minimize side effects overall. If a child's seizures only occur shortly before or after awakening, for example, the largest or only dose should be given at bedtime. Finally, a drug may simply fail because it is ineffective for the specific child.

If two different drugs given singly fail to control seizures, and a combination of two drugs also fails to control seizures—all at dosages that yield blood levels in the mid to upper therapeutic range—the chance that another drug or combination of drugs will fully control the seizures is less than 25 percent. Before trying other medications, it is often worth consulting with an epilepsy specialist to ensure that the diagnosis and medication selection are correct. If seizures are not easily controllable with medication, it may be worth exploring the possibility of dietary therapy, epilepsy surgery, vagus nerve stimulation, or responsive neurostimulation therapy (which is only approved for individuals age 18 years and older). These treatments are discussed in later chapters.

BLOOD TESTING

Before your child starts any AED, your child's doctor will request blood tests. These initial tests provide baseline results that can then be compared with later blood tests. The pre-AED blood tests measure electrolyte levels (such as sodium and potassium), liver and kidney function, and blood-cell counts. Once a medication is started, new blood tests may be done to determine if abnormalities have arisen in these areas and/or to determine the level of medication in the blood. The value of routine blood tests remains unproven; in some cases, they can interfere with care.

How Often Should Blood Tests Be Done After Starting an AED?

There are two types of blood tests, and the question of whether and when to test depends on which type you're talking about. The first kind of test involves obtaining metabolic information (liver enzymes, sodium level, etc.) and blood-cell counts to screen for very, very rare but potentially life-threatening problems (generally less than 1 per 20,000 children develop one of these) related to taking AEDs. Many doctors recommend at least one test to measure metabolic and blood cell levels after starting on a new medication (in addition to the baseline test before starting medication), but in most cases, routine monitoring is not needed. Additional testing may be required if new problems arise, such as serious infection or bleeding, or if seizures increase for no apparent reason.

The second type of test concerns monitoring the drug's blood level. There are two views on how often to perform this test. One view suggests infrequent testing, based on the theory that doctors should "treat the patient, not the laboratory studies." The other encourages frequent monitoring, considering "more information is better." Many American neurologists share the second view and obtain screening blood and follow-up tests/drug levels more often than European and Canadian neurologists, who simply lower the dose if the child has bothersome side effects and raise it if the child has seizures but tolerates the medication well.

For many patients, there's no reason to monitor blood levels unless unexplained seizures or side effects occur, or if the doctor and parents are not sure that the child is taking the drug as prescribed. As with so many decisions faced by patients with epilepsy and their parents, decisions about blood testing should be individually tailored. We recommend blood tests before and then 2 to 10 weeks after a medication is started. Beyond that, it depends on how the patient is doing and what specific drug the patient is taking. For children who have no seizures and no side effects, tests may be obtained once a year or not at all. For those with ongoing seizures but no side effects, the dosage of medication can be increased without checking the levels. In any case, with children it can be worth checking a level to make sure the child is taking the medication, and to assess issues with absorption, metabolism, or drug interactions that could affect the medication levels.

Blood tests to check drug levels should always be performed at a consistent time of day and consistent time after the last dose of medication was taken. This allows the doctor to compare levels at different dosages. Routine blood levels are best measured when the amount of the drug is at its lowest point, the trough level. This generally corresponds to the time just before the medication is taken. Trough levels can fluctuate up to 15 or 20 percent in children who take the drug on a consistent schedule. These variations reflect changes in the absorption and metabolism of the drug, other medications taken, and handling of the blood specimen at the laboratory. Some AEDs, such as valproate and phenytoin, have more variable levels than other AEDs, such as lamotrigine.

One instance in which it may be necessary to check blood levels is before and after adding or removing another medication (including medications taken for conditions other than epilepsy), due to the possibility of drug interactions, as discussed in the next section.

DRUG INTERACTIONS

The doctor caring for your child should be aware of all the drugs your child is taking, because drug interactions are common and can be dangerous. Drug interactions can decrease blood levels of the antiepileptic or other drug, leading to seizures or other problems. Drug blood levels can also increase as a result of drug interactions, leading to toxicity. Even supplements and alternative therapies can cause problems and should be mentioned to your child's doctor. For example, St. John's wort can lower levels of phenobarbital and phenytoin and limit those drugs' effectiveness. Chamomile may intensify or prolong the effects of phenobarbital. Sedating herbs such as kava, valerian, and passionflower can increase the sedation produced by phenobarbital and benzodiazepines.

No list of drug interactions is all-inclusive, as doctors and pharmacists continue to learn about interactions between existing drugs and new ones. Therefore, it's essential to inform all of your child's doctors and other health care providers who prescribe medication that your child is taking an AED. You should also tell the pharmacist and doctors about any use of over-the-counter medications, because some of them can affect AED levels as well. This interaction can cause seizures in someone who has never had a seizure, or increase seizure frequency in a person with epilepsy. The tables in Appendix C list many of the known drug interactions involving AEDs. Over-the-counter drugs that can provoke seizures are also listed in Appendix C. A Web search can also be helpful, but reliability varies widely on the Internet, so make sure to find trustworthy sources (such as epilepsy.com) and verify information at multiple sites.

AEDs and Birth Control

Some adolescents girls wonder about the effect of birth control pills on their seizures, and possible interactions with AEDs. The good news is that most adolescents with epilepsy can take birth control pills without affecting their seizure control, though a minority will find that they have slightly improved or worsened seizure control after starting the pills. Some AEDs (carbamazepine, oxcarbazepine, phenytoin, phenobarbital, primidone, and topiramate) increase the liver's breakdown, or metabolism, of estrogen and progesterone and reduce the effectiveness of birth control pills and other hormone-based therapies (e.g., Depo-Provera). If an adolescent girl is taking birth control pills and one of these drugs, her treatment of conditions like endometriosis, the regulation of her menstrual cycle, or the pills' contraceptive effect may be impaired.

Breakthrough bleeding between menstrual periods is a clue that the effectiveness of birth control pills has been reduced. However, the absence of breakthrough bleeding does not necessarily indicate that the hormonal therapy is fully effective. When taking a hormonal drug and an enzyme-inducing AED such as carbamazepine, patients often find it necessary to use a birth control pill with a higher estrogen content. In these cases, it is wise to also add another method of contraception, such as a barrier device (diaphragm or condom) with spermicide. Clobazam, felbamate, gabapentin, lamotrigine, levetiracetam, valproate, and vigabatrin do not interact significantly with birth control pills. However, felbamate and valproate may increase hormone levels, and a lower dose of birth control medication may be needed. Also, the lamotrigine level is reduced in adolescent girls taking hormonal agents such as estrogen or progesterone, so the dosage of lamotrigine in these patients usually should be increased.

AEDs and Alcohol

The two major concerns when it comes to alcohol use by adolescents with epilepsy—other than the fact that it is illegal and increases the risk of motor vehicle accidents—are side effects and seizures. The adverse effects that accompany many AEDs (at high doses) are similar to the effects of alcohol, including slurred speech, unsteadiness, dizziness, and tiredness. These effects can be exaggerated and thus especially dangerous when people who take AEDs drink alcohol. In addition, consuming more than two alcoholic beverages per 24 hours may lead to withdrawal (most likely to happen four to 48 hours after drinking), during which time seizures are more likely to occur. Drinking more than two alcoholic beverages is also often associated with missing doses of AEDs and sleep deprivation. The combination of these risk factors for seizures—missed doses, alcohol withdrawal, and sleep deprivation—can provoke unusually intense or prolonged seizures.

Also, though alcohol does not seriously alter the effectiveness of AEDs, it can alter the blood levels of patients using some of them. For example, moderate or large alcohol consumption in a short period of time can increase blood phenytoin levels. Prolonged use of alcohol can decrease blood levels of phenobarbital and phenytoin by increasing metabolism.

DISCONTINUING AEDS

Getting their children off AEDs is the goal for most doctors and parents of kids who have well-controlled seizures. Because the majority of children outgrow epilepsy, most are able to easily stop their drug therapy at some point. The question is, when is it best to do so? For children with recurrent seizures, most doctors consider discontinuing AEDs after a seizure-free period of one to two years. Good prognostic factors for coming off medications and staying seizure-free include: (a) few seizures before taking AEDs, (b) seizures were easily controlled with one drug, and (c) normal results on the neurological examination, magnetic resonance imaging (MRI), and EEG.

With certain syndromes, such as benign rolandic epilepsy, it's almost certain that seizures will not recur after age 16, even if medication is discontinued. By contrast, the seizures in JME are often well controlled with medication, but tend to return if the medication is stopped.

COMPOUNDING

Before there were large drug companies, pharmacists routinely combined or processed different ingredients to make a "compounded drug" suited to a specific patient or condition. Though less common, compounding pharmacies are still around and can be helpful in preparing special preparations such as a specially flavored elixir for a drug that is only available as a tablet or in an elixir that the child refuses to swallow. In other cases, a child may be allergic to a "drug" but the allergy is actually to another compound used by the pharmaceutical company in their manufacture of the drug.

MANAGING THE COST OF AEDS

Generic Drugs: A Good Idea?

AEDs are increasingly becoming available in generic form, and the use of these generics is rising, largely because they are less expensive and many insurance companies aren't willing to cover the higher-priced brand-name drugs if generic forms are available. For the vast majority of patients, generics are as effective and safe as brand-name medications. However, some generics are not fully equivalent to the brand-name preparations. The major difference between generic and brand-name medication is not the quality of the drug itself, but rather the consistency in the amount of medication and the way in which it is made. Brand-name drugs are manufactured by major pharmaceutical companies. Generic drugs tend to be made by smaller companies, although this isn't always the case. The manufacturing process can affect how much of the drug is absorbed and the rate at which it is absorbed. The absorption of generic AEDs may be more variable than brand-name drugs. For a small fraction of patients, generic drugs may be associated with greater fluctuations in blood drug levels, leading to a potential increase in seizure frequency (low levels of the drug) and an increase in side effects (high levels).

The FDA requires that the total amount of a generic medication per liquid volume, pill, or capsule—as well as the bioavailability (amount that's absorbed) of the drug—be very similar to the brand-name medication. Even so, there are rare cases where the change from a brand-name drug to a generic drug has led to seizures or side effects; in such cases, with appropriate documentation, insurance companies will usually pay for the patient to take the brand name. If the child's doctor indicates a brand-name drug, the parent may be responsible for paying the difference between the cost of the brand name and the generic, which can be more than $250 per month for one drug. Parents should always check their AEDs before leaving the pharmacy and question the pharmacist if the liquid or pills look different.

Other Ways to Cut Costs

AEDs can be expensive, but there are several ways to cut their costs. Larger-dose forms of drugs often cost only slightly more than lower doses. As a result, it is often cheaper to have the doctor prescribe 200 mg pills and have your child take a half-pill for each dose rather than a full 100 mg pill. Not all pills can be cut, though, so check with the doctor or pharmacist. When choosing health insurance, find out if there is a prescription plan and, if so, how the plan works. Compare the possible increased costs of a health care plan that includes partial or complete coverage for medications to the costs of the drugs, as well as the other benefits.

Before purchasing medication, shop around. You may find a considerable price difference between small pharmacies, large chain stores, mail-order, and Internet plans. Pharmacy services can also help. Most major manufacturers of brand-name AEDs offer assistance programs to make the drugs available to patients with limited incomes (http://www.epilepsy.com/get-help/services-and-support/patient-assistance).

FREQUENTLY ASKED QUESTIONS

How exact do I need to be with the timing of my child's medication? If I give it to my daughter an hour late, could it cause a seizure?

For most patients, taking a medication within two hours of the regular time will not cause seizures or side effects. Indeed, even a single missed dose of medication is unlikely to cause a seizure—but it does significantly increase the risk. Being consistent about the timing of medication helps you avoid missed doses that can lead to seizures, and also helps prevent side effects that may occur when doses are too close together. In general, having a system in place that promotes regular use—for example, taking medications with breakfast and when brushing teeth in the evening—is the best course of action.

My child gets a look on his face that lets me know a seizure is coming on. Can I give him an extra pill when I see that look, and prevent the seizure?

This approach (giving an extra dose in anticipation of a seizure) may work to prevent the seizure, but often it doesn't. That's because in most cases where a child experiences an aura, progression to a larger seizure occurs in mere seconds or a few minutes—not enough time for most oral medicines to reach the brain and take effect. This approach does tend to work, however, in children who are vulnerable to that pending seizure over the coming hours rather than minutes. For example, in a child who has a consistent preseizure sign (such as increased irritability or a headache) 30 to 60 minutes before each episode, a more rapidly acting medicine such as dissolvable clonazepam or oral lorazepam may prevent the seizure. In cases where a seizure is only minutes away, nasal midazolam can be effective in blocking the seizure. The greatest challenge is accuracy—how good are children and parents at predicting when a seizure may occur? If parents over predict and medicate their child when a seizure wouldn't have actually occurred, the child may end up overmedicated and suffer side effects for no necessary reason. Overuse of rescue medication can also lead to the child becoming less sensitive to these medications, or relying too heavily on them—leading to seizures when the medications are withdrawn.

My child started a new AED and is having side effects. Do I need to talk to the doctor about these side effects, or can we just try to wait them out?

It's not unusual to hope that if you ignore something, it will go away. We all do that, but in the case of AED side effects, it is important to hold that impulse at bay. It's true that common side effects such as dizziness or tiredness that occur shortly after a medication is started are often transient and mild. But you should report any more unusual symptoms to your doctor, especially in the first eight weeks after starting a new AED. For example, a new fever or rash could be a serious side effect and may require the doctor to stop the new AED.

If my child stays on her medication for five or 10 years, won't it eventually destroy her liver or kidneys?

No! AEDs do not slowly and progressively damage the liver, like long-term alcohol abuse does.

Can a child's seizures actually get worse from seizure medication?

AEDs can occasionally worsen seizures (Table 9.1). The best protection against this is to keep a log of your child's medication dosage and seizures. If the log indicates that an increase in dosage is associated with an increase in seizures, the doctor should be notified. Be careful not to make false associations, since many factors can contribute to a varying of seizure frequency, and sometimes the reasons remain unknown. For example, a patient or doctor may associate low doses of a new medicine with an increased seizure frequency, when the increase is actually coincidental or the result of lowering another medication. In this instance, the medicine may be very effective for the patient, but the dosage is actually too low rather than too high.

My child has been taking her medication for years. I don't think she's had any side effects, but could I be wrong?

If a child has been on a drug for years, it is often impossible for parents or the child to recognize and assess its side effects. Sometimes the first indication comes when a medication is withdrawn slowly and the child's intellect and mood improve, even though "no problem" was recognized when he was on the medication. It seems that parents' perceptions of cognitive side effects lessen over time more than their perceptions of physical side effects. We may be more likely to accommodate to slowed mental function than a stomachache or blurred vision.

There are also cases where a child or parent *does* report cognitive side effects of an AED, but what they're actually noticing is an effect that instead results primarily from seizures or depression.

The patient, family, and doctor must therefore be vigilant on two fronts: (a) in identifying cognitive impairment resulting from AEDs (especially certain AEDs and high doses or polytherapy), as well as (b) identifying depression. Integrating objective measures of cognitive performance, such as school grades, input from relatives, neuropsychological testing, tracking of seizure frequency relative to cognitive complaints, and assessment of mood can help clarify the underlying cause(s).

Can my child become addicted to medication?

The answer to this question is almost always "No!" In the vast majority of cases, AEDs have no addictive potential. The only AEDs with addictive potential are benzodiazepines (clobazam, clonazepam, clorazepate, and lorazepam) and barbiturates (phenobarbital, primidone). And even addiction to benzodiazepines or barbiturates is rare—it does not occur in children and is very uncommon in adolescents with epilepsy. However, tolerance to these drugs is common; that is, their effect diminishes and higher doses may be needed to achieve the same degree of seizure control.

Benzodiazepines and barbiturates can be successfully discontinued, but this must be done gradually to avoid seizures and other withdrawal symptoms such as rapid heart rate and anxiety. Some withdrawal symptoms occur even when the drug is tapered gradually, especially if the medication has been used for a long time.

According to our doctor, my child's seizure was the result of him missing a medication dose. But how can this be? He's missed many doses in the past, and never seized as a result.

Sometimes a parent will insist that a child has missed doses of medications often, and assumes that thus a breakthrough seizure can't be related to the missed dose. Remember: Missing a dose is gambling. While the odds may be small that a seizure will occur from a single missed dose of medication, if the omission is repeated regularly, the chances increase that a seizure will result. Another way to think of this is that without AED treatment, seizures do not occur every day. Your child may benefit from AEDs only a few days a year, but you can't tell which days these might be. Miss a dose on a nonseizure day, no problem. Miss a dose on a seizure day, and a seizure is not prevented.

You will almost certainly have questions of your own as you consider drug therapy for your child—and during the therapy itself, if prescribed. The doctor, nurses, and pharmacist who work with your family can answer your questions. Keep an eye out for any changes that your child goes through while starting medication, and keep notes if necessary, so that you can talk about these changes and any associated questions with your child's team. The idea of drug therapy can seem daunting and complicated, but AEDs have become a very common and safe treatment for children with epilepsy, a treatment that often allows these children to lead full lives alongside their peers.

10 DRUGS USED FOR TREATING EPILEPSY

Selecting the right antiepileptic drug for your child is a complex process in which your doctor will take into account your child's seizure type and epilepsy syndrome, the likely effectiveness and possible side effects of the drug, other benefits of the drug (such as weight loss or preventing migraines), the potential of the drug to make some types of seizures worse, any possible problems that might accompany the drug (weight gain, tiredness), cost, how often the drug must be taken, and possible interactions. Your doctor will also factor in any scientific data that's available from controlled trials, local medical practices, his or her own experience, and the family's input. This chapter reviews the most frequently used antiepileptic drugs (AEDs) and also some experimental ones; the characteristics of the different AEDs are summarized in Table 10.1, and their side effects are summarized in Table 10.2. Appendix C lists the major interactions that these drugs have with other medications.

TABLE 10.1: CHARACTERISTICS OF FREQUENTLY USED ANTIEPILEPTIC DRUGS WHEN USED ALONE

Drug	Average Daily Dose (mg/kg) for Children*	Time to Peak Blood Level[a] (hr)	Therapeutic Blood Levels (mcg/mL of blood)	Half-life[b] (hr)
Acetazolamide	8–30	2–4	10–30	10–12
Carbamazepine[c]	<6 y-o: 15–35 mg 6–12 y-o: <1,000 mg	2–12	5–12	6–22
Clonazepam[d]	0.1–0.2	1–4	20–80 (ng/mL)	15–50
Clorazepate	3.75–15 mg	0.5–2	Unknown	30–100

(continued)

TABLE 10.1: CHARACTERISTICS OF FREQUENTLY USED ANTIEPILEPTIC DRUGS WHEN USED ALONE (*CONTINUED*)

Drug	Average Daily Dose (mg/kg) for Children*	Time to Peak Blood Level[a] (hr)	Therapeutic Blood Levels (mcg/mL of blood)	Half-life[b] (hr)
Ethosuximide[d]	3–6 y-o: 20–30 mg >6 y-o: 500–1,000 mg	1–4	50–100	25–70
Felbamate[d]	15–45	1–4	30–100	14–20
Gabapentin[d]	25–50	2–4	4–16	5–7
Lamotrigine[d]	2–8	2–4	2–14	7–60[g]
Levetiracetam	10–40	1–2	15–55	6–8
Oxcarbazepine	6–50	3–6	10–35**	10
Perampanel	Uncertain (~0.1–0.25)	0.5–3	?200–400 ng/ml	100
Phenobarbital	2–8	2–12	12–40	26–140
Phenytoin	4–7	4–8	10–20	14–30[h]
Pregabalin	3–8	1–3	1–10	4–7
Primidone	<25	2–5	5–18	12
Tiagabine	0.5–2	1–2	5–70 mg/mL	4–9
Topiramate	3–9	2–4	2–25	20
Valproate[d]	15–60	2–8 1–3[i]	50–120	8–15
Zonisamide	2–12	5–6	10–40	40–60

mg, milligram (one thousandth of a gram); mcg, microgram (one millionth of a gram); ng, nanogram (one billionth of a gram); y-o, year old.

* Actual doses used can vary considerably, as some patients may be seizure-free at lower doses and others may require and tolerate higher doses. When used in combination with other drugs, dosages may vary.

** MHD, active metabolite, is measured.

[a] After drug blood levels reach steady state; may reflect sustained-release preparation.

[b] Children metabolize many drugs more rapidly than adults do, so the half-life is often shorter in children.

[c] Active metabolite.

[d] In general, when these drugs are given together with carbamazepine, phenobarbital, phenytoin, or primidone, their blood level is lower and their half-life is shorter.

[g] Valproate prolongs the half-life of lamotrigine.

[h] The half-life of phenytoin increases as the dose or blood level increase.

[i] After oral dose of valproate.

TABLE 10.2: MAJOR ADVERSE EFFECTS OF DRUGS COMMONLY USED TO TREAT EPILEPSY

Drug	Dose-Related Side Effects[a]	Rare Idiosyncratic Side Effects	Long-Term Side Effects
Acetazolamide	Increased frequency of urination, tingling of face, fingers, toes	Kidney stones	None
Benzodiazepines Clobazam Clonazepam Clorazepate Diazepam Lorazepam	Tiredness, dizziness, unsteadiness, impaired attention and memory, hyperactivity, depression, irritability, aggressivity, drooling (children), nausea, loss of appetite	Extremely rare—Low platelets or blood cells	None
Carbamazepine Eslicarbazepine Oxcarbazepine	Nausea, vomiting, blurred or double vision, tiredness, dizziness, unsteadiness, poor coordination, impotence, memory problems, slurred speech, low sodium (hyponatremia; uncommon), tremor, weight gain, fever[b]	Rash (~4%) Rare—Severe rash Very rare for carbamazepine and oxcarbazepine— Very low blood cell counts (bone marrow suppression), liver damage, heart block (a blockage of electrical impulses in the heart)	Bone loss
Ethosuximide	Nausea and vomiting, loss of appetite, weight loss, behavioral changes, tiredness, dizziness, earache	Very low blood cell counts (bone marrow suppression)	None
Felbamate	Headache, insomnia, irritability, nausea, vomiting, weight loss	Bone marrow or liver failure (combined risk estimated at about 1 in 4,500), rash, severe rash	None

(continued)

TABLE 10.2: MAJOR ADVERSE EFFECTS OF DRUGS COMMONLY USED TO TREAT EPILEPSY (*CONTINUED*)

Drug	Dose-Related Side Effects[a]	Rare Idiosyncratic Side Effects	Long-Term Side Effects
Gabapentin	Dizziness, tiredness, weight gain, leg swelling	None	None
Lamotrigine	Insomnia, nausea, unsteadiness blurred/double vision	Severe rash	None
Levetiracetam	Tiredness, dizziness, unsteadiness, irritability	Unknown	Unknown
Mephobarbital Phenobarbital Primidone	Tiredness, depression, hyperactivity, dizziness, memory problems, impotence, slurred speech, nausea, anemia, low calcium levels, bone loss	Liver damage, severe rash, hypersensitivity reaction Infrequent—rash	Bone loss, soft tissue growths, rheumatological disorders (frozen shoulder, stiffening of fingers)
Perampanel	Tiredness, dizziness, headache, irritability, anxiety, depression	Serious psychiatric disorders; may be primarily dose-related	None known
Phenytoin	Tiredness, dizziness, memory problems, rash or fever, gum overgrowth, growth of facial hair, anemia, acne, slurred speech, low calcium, bone loss	Liver damage, severe and other hypersensitivity reactions, behavioral changes Infrequent—rash	Bone loss, nerve damage, possible damage to cerebellum (part of brain)
Pregabalin	Dizziness, tiredness, behavioral change, weight gain	None	None
Tiagabine	Dizziness, tiredness, mood changes	Status epilepticus	None
Topiramate	Dizziness, tiredness, decreased appetite, impaired concentration and word finding, memory problems, mood changes	Kidney stones, rash, glaucoma, heat stroke (in children)	None

(*continued*)

TABLE 10.2: MAJOR ADVERSE EFFECTS OF DRUGS COMMONLY USED TO TREAT EPILEPSY (*CONTINUED*)

Drug	Dose-Related Side Effects[a]	Rare Idiosyncratic Side Effects	Long-Term Side Effects
Valproate	Nausea and vomiting, tiredness, weight gain, hair loss, tremor	Liver damage, very low platelet counts, pancreatic inflammation, hearing loss, behavioral changes	Bone loss, hair loss, hair texture change, weight gain
Vigabatrin	Tiredness, weight gain	None	Damage to retina of eye and impairment of peripheral vision
Zonisamide	Drowsiness, dizziness, loss of appetite, GI discomfort	Kidney stones, rash	Possible bone loss

WBC, white blood cell count; CBC, complete blood cell count; GI, gastrointestinal.

[a]*Some of the side effects (very low blood cell or platelet count, liver damage, hypersensitivity reactions, severe rash, pancreatic inflammation) are serious and potentially fatal.*

A NOTE ON FDA (FOOD AND DRUG ADMINISTRATION) APPROVAL

Most of the drugs mentioned in this chapter are approved by the Food and Drug Administration (FDA), but not all are approved specifically for primary treatment of all epilepsy syndromes. This is partly a function of the way that FDA approval works. The approval process requires that specific study designs be completed before a drug can receive an indication from the FDA (an *indication* means that the drug has been approved as treatment for a particular disease or syndrome). There are three areas in epilepsy where doctors commonly prescribe outside of FDA indications: pediatrics, generalized epilepsy, and monotherapy.

Pediatrics and generalized epilepsy: Most AEDs are studied mainly or exclusively in adults with focal epilepsy. The leap from adults to children in relation to these drugs is small: The drugs that are effective for adults with focal epilepsy are effective for children with focal epilepsy. However, children can have different drug-metabolism and side-effect profiles than adults.

The leap from focal epilepsy to generalized epilepsy isn't so direct. In some cases, drugs for focal epilepsy can actually increase the frequency or severity of generalized seizures. However, other drugs approved initially for focal epilepsy are also effective for treating generalized epilepsy (lamotrigine, levetiracetam, perampanel, topiramate) and have subsequently received FDA approval to do so. Still others (felbamate and zonisamide) appear effective in many patients with generalized epilepsy, but they do not yet have an FDA indication for this disorder. Your doctor may prescribe these drugs based on their record of effectiveness in other patients, even though they don't have an FDA indication for your child's syndrome.

In the case of *monotherapy*: Until recently, for a drug to receive a monotherapy indication for epilepsy, studies had to prove that that drug was more effective than a placebo. That has recently changed, and now a drug only has to show equivalence to an established, effective AED (proof that the second drug's clinical effect is equal to the first's) in order to receive a monotherapy indication. This is great news, since it's traditionally been hard to get AEDs approved for monotherapy. Parents or patients who consent for drug studies are usually those with very difficult-to-control focal seizures that haven't been alleviated by approved AEDs. However, it is dangerous and unethical to take someone who has seizures on effective medications and randomize them to either a new drug (which may not be effective) or placebo. As a result, most new drugs are tested in "add-on" or adjunctive studies: Patients on an existing drug therapy are randomized to receive an additional new drug or placebo. Such studies can result only in an adjunctive ("add-on") indication for the new drug from the FDA, but not a monotherapy indication. These challenges, as well as expense, lead many companies to settle for the adjunctive indication, knowing that many doctors and nurse practitioners (like us) would still prescribe the AED as monotherapy based on the clinical situation.

Overall, FDA indications are a conservative guide when it comes to prescribing AEDs and may not always serve your child's best interests. If a drug is effective and well tolerated, but only indicated in adults as adjunctive therapy, many epilepsy experts will use it in children or as monotherapy. Caution is needed in using a drug approved only for focal epilepsy for those with generalized epilepsy. However, if other medications are ineffective or intolerable, and anecdotal data strongly suggests effectiveness, a trial may be considered. Regardless of the specific therapy, the parents and doctor must jointly assess its benefits and side effects—even drugs used within an FDA indication may be ineffective or occasionally exacerbate seizures.

A NOTE ON SIDE EFFECTS

All AEDs have the potential to cause side effects. In general, the higher the dosage and the greater number of AEDs the child is on, the more likely it is that side effects will occur. Many parents read the list of side effects (Table 10.2) or more extensive lists on the Internet that include rare to exceedingly rare side effects and understandably fear that the risks of an AED far outweigh the benefits. This is usually not true when an AED is recommended by a doctor. You should understand the common side effects—those that occur in more than 5 percent of children (over the rate of the problem when children were given placebos in drug trials)—as well as the less common but potentially serious side effects such as rash.

Many side effects are common to multiple AEDs, such as tiredness, dizziness, or nausea. They usually improve with time or can be reduced by adjusting the timing or amount of medication and their relationship to meals. In some cases, the side effects are more troublesome and the doctor should be notified. When your child starts an AED, it is not a long-term commitment—it is a trial process to determine if the drug is effective and well tolerated. If not, other AEDs can be tried.

For the rare side effects, think risk versus benefit. Many parents read about the potentially life-threatening rash that can occur with lamotrigine and feel that this is a medication they would never want their child to take. Yet for most epilepsy doctors, it is one of the first medications they would choose for themselves or their child. This is because it is effective for many seizure types and, for the vast majority of children and adults, very well tolerated. If the dose is gradually increased, the risk of the life-threatening rash is one in 20,000 and the risk of dying is lower. For the average American child or adult, there is a one in 7,000 chance every year of dying in a car accident. Similarly, for children with treatment-resistant epilepsy, many parents read about the potentially fatal bone marrow or liver failure associated with felbamate and decide never to use this drug. Yet with regular blood tests during the first year of use, the risk of death is less than one in 10,000 (likely less than one in 20,000). For adolescents with treatment-resistant epilepsy, the risk from dying from epilepsy may be more than 5 percent per decade. It is hard, but try to take emotion out of these decisions.

DRUGS COMMONLY USED AGAINST EPILEPSY

The following pages discuss the most commonly used AEDs, listed alphabetically. A discussion of the role of benzodiazepines (clonazepam, clobazam, clorazepate, diazepam, lorazepam) follows at the end of the chapter (see page 133). Table 10.1 summarizes many features of specific AEDs, such as their dosage, time to peak blood level, therapeutic range, and half-life; Table 10.2 summarizes their side effects.

Acetazolamide

Acetazolamide (Diamox®) can be used in combination with another drug to treat absence and myoclonic seizures. It is also used to treat focal or generalized seizures that occur around menstruation (catamenial epilepsy). Acetazolamide inhibits the enzyme carbonic anhydrase. Proof of its long-term effectiveness in epilepsy is limited; the drug may become less effective over time. Side effects are usually mild and include dizziness; tingling of the lips, fingertips, and toes; and increased urination (acetazolamide is a mild diuretic). About 1 to 2 percent of patients taking it on a regular basis develop kidney stones, so children using the drug should drink plenty of fluids, especially when in hot environments or with vigorous or prolonged exercise. The ketogenic diet (see Chapter 11), topiramate, and zonisamide can also predispose to kidney stones, and so acetazolamide should be used cautiously with these therapies.

Acetazolamide is available in 125 mg and 250 mg tablets. There is no clearly defined therapeutic range of drug blood levels. Acetazolamide is also used to prevent altitude sickness.

Carbamazepine

Carbamazepine (Tegretol®, Tegretol-XR®, Carbatrol®) is a first-line drug for all types of focal seizures and focal epilepsy syndromes. The liver metabolizes this drug more rapidly after a person has been taking it for several weeks. Common side effects include tiredness, blurry or double vision, nausea, dizziness, and unsteadiness. Rash occurs in approximately 5 percent of patients on the drug and is much more common in Asian patients with the HLA-B*1502 gene variant. Asian patients should be screened for this gene. Decreased vitamin D levels and bone loss may follow long-term use. Very rare (<1/25,000 patients) life-threatening side effects are liver failure and bone marrow failure. Carbamazepine can lower the amount of sodium in the blood and can cause mild weight gain.

Carbamazepine is available as a generic and brand name (Tegretol® and Carbatrol®) drug in various strengths: chewable 100 mg and regular 200 mg tablets, and a liquid elixir (100 mg per teaspoon). Extended-release tablets are also available in 100, 200, 300, and 400 mg sizes. In some forms of the extended release, the pill's shell, which is not absorbed, has a small hole in it that slowly releases the medication. There is no need to worry if the shell is found in the stool; the medicine has been absorbed. Carbamazepine is also used to stabilize mood in patients with bipolar disorder and to reduce pain due to nerve, spinal cord, or brain disorders.

Eslicarbazepine

Eslicarbazepine acetate (Aptiom®) is approved for monotherapy and adjunctive therapy of focal onset seizures in adults. Eslicarbazepine acetate is a prodrug (a compound that is inactive or not fully active when administered) that is rapidly metabolized into eslicarbazepine, which is also the active metabolite of oxcarbazepine. Thus, both eslicarbazepine acetate and oxcarbazepine work using the same active metabolite, which inhibits fast-conducting sodium channels. One benefit of eslicarbazepine acetate over oxcarbazepine is that it produces lower peak levels of eslicarbazepine, and thus is associated with fewer side effects. Side effects are similar to those of oxcarbazepine and carbamazepine, and include tiredness, dizziness, headache, blurred or double vision, unsteadiness, rash, and low blood sodium.

Although not approved for use in children, this drug may be used in children who can swallow pills. Pediatric dosing of eslicarbazepine acetate is not established, but our experience is that 12 to 20 mg/kg doses are often effective and well tolerated. Aptiom is available as 200, 400, 600, and 800 mg doses. Eslicarbazepine can also be used to treat bipolar disorder and trigeminal neuralgia.

Ethosuximide

Ethosuximide (Zarontin®) is used to treat only absence seizures. It is not effective in treating other generalized seizures (myoclonic, tonic–clonic) or focal seizures. It works by blocking certain calcium channels in the brain. It is usually well tolerated, but side effects can include nausea and vomiting, loss of appetite, weight loss, behavioral changes, tiredness, and dizziness. The recommended pediatric dose is approximately 20 mg/kg. Ethosuximide is available as a 250 mg gelcap (amber) or a liquid elixir (250 mg/5 mL).

Ezogabine (Retigabine)

Ezogabine (Potiga®) is approved for adjunctive therapy of focal epilepsies in adults; data on its pediatric use is limited. Ezogabine's mechanism of action is unique: It opens potassium channels in the brain. Anecdotal data suggests it is helpful in epilepsies associated with Ring chromosome 20. The most common side effects are drowsiness, dizziness, and unsteadiness. Less common side effects include rash, cognitive impairment, behavioral changes, and tremors. Although uncommon, ezogabine can cause blue skin discoloration, pigment changes in the retina, and impaired urination—these side effects have limited more widespread use. It has a half-life of 8 to 10 hours, and is often given three times a day. Potiga is available as 50, 200, 300, and 400 mg immediate-release tablets.

Felbamate

Felbamate (Felbatol®) is effective in treating focal and secondarily generalized tonic–clonic seizures and Lennox–Gastaut syndrome, and may also help control generalized seizures, but is in limited use (see later in this section). The drug is usually given two to three times daily. It is generally well tolerated, and some patients report feeling "more awake" or "brighter" on it. Common side effects are decreased appetite, weight loss, insomnia, and headache. Uncommon and usually mild side effects include cognitive and behavioral problems. Rash is possible. Pediatric doses range from 15 to 45 mg/kg. Felbamate (Felbatol®) is available as an elixir (600 mg/5 mL; fruit punch flavor) and in 400 mg (yellow) and 600 mg (peach) tablets. Generic forms are also available.

Important note: When felbamate was in greater use, and before blood tests were carefully monitored, the drug had an approximately 1 in 4,500 risk of bone marrow failure or liver failure that was fatal in approximately half of affected individuals (approximately 1 in 9,000 died). Its use is now strictly limited to patients in whom the benefits outweigh the risks. Blood cell counts and liver-function tests should be performed often (every two weeks is recommended), at least during the first year of therapy, which is when most of the serious problems occur. (See previous note on side effects.)

Gabapentin

Gabapentin (Neurontin®) is effective for all focal seizures but ineffective for all generalized seizures. Even with focal seizures, gabapentin is considered less effective than some other drugs. It's approved for adjunctive use, but it can be effective in monotherapy for select patients. Gabapentin is an amino acid chemically related to the inhibitory neurotransmitter gamma-amino butyric acid (GABA), but it does not work like GABA and its precise mechanism of action is unknown. It has a short half-life of approximately six hours and is usually taken two to three times a day, although longer-acting once-daily preparations (Gralise®) are available. Most children take doses of approximately 25 to 50 mg/kg/d in two or three divided doses.

Gabapentin is usually very well tolerated. The most common side effects are dose-related tiredness and dizziness, which often improve after several weeks. Other side effects include headache, unsteadiness, visual changes, abdominal discomfort, edema (swelling) in the limbs (especially feet), and weight gain. Behavioral problems such as irritability and hyperactivity can occur in children, although gabapentin can also improve the patient's mood. Gabapentin does not cause life-threatening side effects.

Gabapentin is excreted unchanged in the urine. The lack of liver metabolism and protein binding means that it does not interact with other drugs. Gabapentin is available as a generic (capsule and tablet) and also as brand-name Neurontin® in hard gelatin capsules that carry doses of 100 mg (white), 300 mg (yellow), and 400 mg (orange), and in scored tablets of 600 mg and 800 mg (white ovals). Long-acting Gralise® comes in 300 and 600 mg tablets. An elixir (250 mg/5 mL) is also available. Gabapentin is also beneficial in treating some headache and pain syndromes.

Lacosamide

Lacosamide (Vimpat®) is approved as monotherapy and adjunctive (add-on) therapy for the treatment of all focal seizures in individuals over age 17. Like many other AEDs, it works on the sodium channel, but whereas other AEDs (e.g., carbamazepine, lamotrigine) affect the fast inactivation mechanism, lacosamide affects the slow inactivation mechanism. We do not fully understand the therapeutic implications of these differential effects on the inactivation of sodium channels. It is rapidly absorbed and has a half-life of about 14 hours. It is usually given twice daily. The most common side effects are dizziness, unsteadiness, blurred or double vision, and nausea. Less common side effects are vomiting and impaired cognition. Lacosamide is only available as a brand-name (Vimpat®) drug and comes in 50 mg (pink), 100 mg (dark yellow), 150 mg (salmon), and 200 mg (blue) tablets. It is also available as a 10 mg/mL syrup. Children are often started on doses of about 1 mg/kg/d and increased to a target dose of 3 to 10 mg/kg day as needed and tolerated.

Lamotrigine

Lamotrigine (Lamictal®) is effective in treating all focal seizures, generalized absence and tonic–clonic seizures, and Lennox–Gastaut syndrome. It can be used alone or as adjunctive therapy. Its approximately 24-hour half-life is affected by other AEDs: roughly doubled by valproate and halved by drugs that induce liver enzymes (e.g., carbamazepine, phenytoin). Lamotrigine levels may be decreased by contraceptive pills and patches. Lamotrigine is given once or twice a day (especially in patients taking drugs that induce liver enzymes). Pediatric dosages start at 0.6 mg/kg/d in two divided doses for one to two weeks, then increase to 1.2 mg/kg/d, and finally are increased weekly to reach a dose of 5 to 10 mg/kg/d as a single therapy. Children who can swallow pills may be given a long-acting form once daily.

Lamotrigine is generally well tolerated; in some patients, energy, mood, and emotional well-being improve. Side effects include dizziness, unsteadiness, blurred vision, headache, nausea, diarrhea, insomnia, tiredness, and rash. The frequency and severity of the rash are greater if the dosage is increased rapidly. The rash usually involves the trunk, arms, or face, and is more likely in patients who also take valproate. A potentially life-threatening rash (known as Stevens–Johnson syndrome) can develop, especially in children on valproate in whom the dose is increased rapidly. Lamotrigine should be started at a very low dosage and increased very gradually, especially if the patient is taking valproate. Though this slow titration is important because of the rash issues, it's a therapeutic disadvantage, since the slow start means it can take a month or two for the drug's therapeutic benefits to take effect.

Lamotrigine is available as 5 mg (chewable), 25 mg (chewable and regular), 100 mg, 150 mg, and 200 mg tablets. Extended-release pills come in 25, 50, 100, 200, 250, and 300 mg dosages. There are currently no capsule or liquid forms available. Generic forms of the chewable, immediate-release, and extended-release compounds are available. Lamotrigine is also used to treat bipolar disorder.

Important note: Lamisil®—an antifungal drug—has occasionally been mistakenly given instead of Lamictal®, so always read the label!

Levetiracetam

Levetiracetam (Keppra®) is FDA approved as adjunctive therapy for children and adults with focal epilepsy, and also as treatment for myoclonic seizures in patients with juvenile myoclonic epilepsy and generalized tonic–clonic seizures. Its half-life is 7 to 12 hours. The drug is mainly excreted unchanged in the urine; it isn't metabolized in the liver and has no known interactions with other drugs. The most commonly reported side effects are tiredness and behavioral changes. Uncommon side effects include dizziness, nausea, unsteadiness, weakness, insomnia, and headache. Irritability, depression, and aggressive behaviors can occur and are the most common reasons that patients (about 10 percent of children) discontinue the drug. These problems are more common when the dosage is rapidly increased, and also in children and in patients with developmental disabilities. Rash is rare. The pediatric dosage starts at 7 to 10 mg/kg/d, given in two or occasionally three doses. This dosage is increased as tolerated and needed over two to six weeks, up to a maximum of 45 to 60 mg/kg/d.

Levetiracetam is available as 250 mg, 500 mg, 750 mg, and 1,000 mg tablets; the extended-release tablets come in 500 mg and 750 mg sizes. This drug is also available as an elixir (100 mg/mL) and for intravenous use. Generic forms are available.

Oxcarbazepine

Oxcarbazepine (Trileptal®, Oxtellar XR®) is closely chemically related to carbamazepine. It is FDA approved as monotherapy and adjunctive therapy for treating focal seizures in children and adults. Its side effect profile is similar to that of carbamazepine, with the main effects being tiredness, dizziness, headache, blurred or double vision, and unsteadiness. Among patients in whom carbamazepine causes a rash, about 25 percent will have a rash when later treated with oxcarbazepine. Like carbamazepine, the drug has infrequent cognitive side effects. The level of sodium in the blood may become low (hyponatremia), which is usually asymptomatic but may occasionally cause tiredness, dizziness, and increased seizure frequency. Decreased vitamin D levels and bone loss may follow long-term use.

The half-life of oxcarbazepine is about two hours, but its antiseizure effect comes from the formation of an active byproduct (monohydroxyderivative, MHD) with a half-life of 10 hours. Oxcarbazepine is available as Trileptal® and Oxtellar XR®, each in three sizes: 150 mg, 300 mg, and 600 mg. It is also offered as an oral suspension (300 mg/5 mL). Generic forms are also available.

Perampanel

Perampanel (Fycompa®) is approved for the adjunctive treatment of focal and primary generalized tonic–clonic seizures in patients with epilepsy 12 years of age and older. Perampanel is a noncompetitive AMPA receptor antagonist that blocks the effect of glutamate, the main excitatory neurotransmitter in the brain. The most common side effects are dizziness, somnolence, headache, fatigue, and behavioral changes. Doses of up to 12 mg/d are used in adults. Enzyme-inducing AEDs (e.g., carbamazepine) lower the blood level of perampanel. No dose recommendations are available in children under age 12. Perampanel is available as 2 mg, 4 mg, 6 mg, 8 mg, 10 mg, and 12 mg tablets.

Phenobarbital

Phenobarbital is one of the oldest AEDs and is used to treat focal seizures, generalized tonic–clonic seizures, and neonatal seizures. Phenobarbital's long half-life can range from 60 to 180 hours. It is often given once a day. The dosage in children usually ranges from 3 to 5 mg/kg/d (slightly higher, 5–8 mg/kg, for children ages two months to two years). Phenobarbital works by enhancing the effects of the inhibitory neurotransmitter GABA.

Common side effects include tiredness, hyperactivity, dizziness, unsteadiness, cognitive impairments, depression, and rash. Phenobarbital induces the liver enzyme (cytochrome P450) system and often lowers the levels of other medications by stimulating their metabolism. This effect also increases the metabolism of vitamin D and may contribute to the development of bone loss (osteopenia, osteoporosis). Long-term use of phenobarbital can also cause soft-tissue changes including fibrosis of ligaments, frozen shoulder, and knuckle and heel pads. Phenobarbital is available as pills (16.2 mg, 32.4 mg, and 64.8 mg) and an elixir (20 mg/5 mL).

Phenytoin

Phenytoin (Dilantin®, Phenytek®) is a first-line drug for all types of focal seizures. The daily dose ranges from 6 to 10 mg/kg/d, with higher doses in infants and young children, due to their higher metabolism. In emergency settings, it (or its prodrug fosphenytoin/Cerebyx®) may be given intravenously to rapidly achieve therapeutic levels. The half-life in children is often less than eight hours, so dosing two to three times a day is recommended unless an extended-release preparation is used.

Side effects include tiredness, dizziness, unsteadiness, slurred speech, acne, rash (6 percent of patients), and darker or excessive hair (hirsutism), which is most troublesome for girls. Cognitive and behavioral problems are infrequent and usually mild at therapeutic blood levels. Long-term use can lower vitamin D levels and cause bone loss, soft-tissue growths, and, rarely, nerve injury (neuropathy) or loss of tissue in the cerebellum of the brain (possibly related to periods of very high blood levels). Because phenytoin can cause gum overgrowth (hyperplasia), maintaining regular dental visits and flossing and brushing are important. Very rare (less than 1 in 100,000) life-threatening side effects include liver failure, bone marrow failure (aplastic anemia), and severe rash.

The metabolism and clearance (rate at which an active drug is cleared from the body) of phenytoin slows as the dose rises. This can cause very slow accumulation and overdose, leading to hospitalization. The amount in the bloodstream may continue to increase for up to a month after a dose change. Conversely, reduction in the dose may lead to unusually large decreases in the blood level that can prompt increased seizure activity. This is an important issue in children and phenytoin is one drug where blood level monitoring is often needed.

Phenytoin is available as a generic 100 mg extended-release capsule. Dilantin® is available as a 30 mg capsule or a 100 mg capsule, or as a 50 mg chewable tablet (Infatab). Phenytek® is available as a 200 and 300 mg capsule. Dilantin® is also available as an elixir (125 mg/5 ml) and as an intravenous preparation, which should only be used in the hospital. Intravenous fosphenytoin (Cerebyx®) is safer because it does not cause serious complications if it leaks out of the vein. Fosphenytoin is rapidly converted into phenytoin by the liver.

Pregabalin

Pregabalin (Lyrica®) is approved as an adjunctive therapy for adults with focal epilepsy. It is closely related to gabapentin, and is also an analogue of GABA. Common side effects include tiredness and dizziness. Tremors, unsteadiness, visual changes, dry mouth, and peripheral edema (swelling) may occur, mainly in the feet. Weight gain can occur with long-term use. There are no known life-threatening side effects.

Pregabalin's half-life is 6 to 10 hours in adults, but data on children is lacking; it is usually dosed twice a day. It is excreted unchanged in the urine and has no drug interactions. Adult doses range from 150 to 600 mg/d; pediatric doses can range from 3 to 8 mg/kg/d. The drug comes in 25, 50, 75, 100, 150, 200, and 300 mg tablets. Pregabalin is also effective in treating neuropathic pain and anxiety disorders.

Rufinamide

Rufinamide (Banzel®) is approved for adjunctive (add-on) treatment of seizures associated with Lennox–Gastaut syndrome in children four years of age and older and adults. Studies also suggest that rufinamide may be helpful in treating focal seizures. Although rufinamide has some effect on sodium channels, its mechanism of antiepilepsy action is largely unknown. The time to peak blood levels is four to six hours. The half-life of rufinamide is 6 to 10 hours. Rufinamide is usually started orally at 10 mg/kg/d, titrating up by 10 mg/kg/d every two to seven days to a target dosage of 45 mg/kg/d divided twice daily (maximum dosage of 3,200 mg/d). Rufinamide is available as 200 mg and 400 mg tablets and as a 40 mg/mL orange-flavored liquid.

Tiagabine

Tiagabine (Gabitril®) is approved for treating focal epilepsy in patients age 12 years and older. It prolongs the action of GABA by blocking its reuptake by cells. Its half-life is approximately five to eight hours. Twice-a-day dosing is effective; however, it's often given three times a day. The dose is often started at 0.25 mg/kg/d and increased to 1 to 1.5 mg/kg/d.

Common side effects include dizziness, tiredness, nervousness, and headache. Occasional side effects are tremor, nausea, diarrhea, weakness, irritability, difficulty concentrating, and confusion. Drug interactions are uncommon, although tiagabine is metabolized more rapidly in patients taking drugs that induce liver enzymes.

Tiagabine is available as 4 mg, 12 mg (green oval), 16 mg, and 20 mg tablets. No capsules or liquids are currently available. Generic 2 mg and 4 mg tiagabine tablets are available.

Topiramate

Topiramate (Topamax®, Trokendi XR®, Qudexy XR®) is approved for monotherapy and adjunctive therapy in patients 10 years or older with focal epilepsy or primary generalized tonic–clonic seizures, and in patients with Lennox–Gastaut syndrome.

Side effects include tiredness, dizziness, unsteadiness, weight loss, constipation, tingling (usually in the fingers, toes, or around the mouth), double vision or other visual problems, problems with concentration, slowing of thought processes, word-finding problems, depression, and irritability. Most children tolerate the drug well when started at a low dose that is increased gradually, but the side effects can be disabling no matter how slowly it is introduced. The extended-release preparations are often better tolerated because of their lower peak-dose side effects. Because topiramate can cause kidney stones in 1 to 2 percent of patients, it should be used cautiously in patients on the ketogenic diet and people taking acetazolamide or zonisamide. Patients should drink adequate fluids, especially in hot environments or with exercise. It can rarely cause glaucoma or inhibit sweating, which may lead to heat stroke in hot weather when fluid intake is inadequate. Topiramate has few significant drug interactions. It can slightly raise phenytoin levels, and drugs that induce liver enzymes (e.g., carbamazepine, phenytoin) can lower topiramate levels by up to 50 percent.

The half-life is approximately 15 hours in children and approximately eight hours in children on enzyme-inducing medications; it is usually given twice a day, unless an extended release form is used. The average daily adult dose ranges from 10 to 40 mg/kg/d.

Topiramate is available as 15 mg and 25 mg sprinkle capsules, as well as 25 mg, 100 mg, and 200 mg tablets. Topiramate extended-release tablets are available in

25 mg, 50 mg, 100 mg, and 200 mg tablets. The tablets are not scored and have a very bitter taste if broken. Extended-release tablets become immediate release if they are crushed or split. No liquid form is available.

Valproate

Valproate (valproic acid; Depakene®, Depakote®/divalproex sodium) is effective in treating all generalized and focal seizure types. It is a first-line drug for treating several generalized epilepsy syndromes (juvenile myoclonic epilepsy, absence epilepsy with tonic–clonic seizures).

Common side effects of valproate limit its use. Both sexes can develop weight gain and hair loss. Girls can develop hormonal disorders such as irregular menses and polycystic ovarian syndrome. If the drug is used during pregnancy, the risk of birth defects goes up significantly, as does the risk of developmental delays in the child. Other common side effects include tiredness, dizziness, nausea, vomiting, and behavioral changes that include depression in adults and irritability in children. Long-term use of valproate can cause bone loss and ankle swelling. Rare and dangerous side effects are liver damage (more common in children under age two years), very low platelet numbers, inflammation of the pancreas, confusion, and hearing loss.

Anecdotal evidence suggests that hair loss and pancreatic inflammation may be prevented or reduced by taking the minerals selenium (10–20 mcg/d) and zinc (25–50 mg/d)—and also biotin for hair loss (10–30 mcg in children under age 10; 30–100 mcg in older children); proof is lacking that these supplements are effective. Many high-potency multivitamins contain these dosages. The risk of life-threatening liver toxicity is very low: approximately one in 50,000 adults and children over two years who take the drug. The highest risk (~1/500) is in children under six months who also take other AEDs.

Valproate is available as a generic drug in 125 mg, 250 mg, and 500 mg tablets and a liquid (200 mg/5 mL). Depakene® (valproate) is available as a 250 mg tablet and in liquid form (250 mg/5 mL). A delayed-release preparation is available as a 125 mg sprinkle capsule and as 125 mg, 250 mg, and 500 mg tablets; the extended release is also offered as divalproex sodium ER (250 mg and 500 mg tablets). Valproate is also an effective preventive therapy for migraine headaches and bipolar disorder when taken every day.

Vigabatrin

Vigabatrin (Sabril®) is used mainly to treat infantile spasms and treatment-resistant focal seizures. Because retinal toxicity is a potential side effect, the drug is not indicated for first-line use in focal epilepsy and is only recommended after a child has failed other AEDs. Vigabatrin is often very effective at treating all seizure types in patients with tuberous sclerosis and may have similar efficacy for children with focal cortical dysplasia. Its half-life is about five to six hours, but its action lasts six days. It is usually taken twice a day.

Vigabatrin typically is well tolerated. Drowsiness and fatigue are the most common side effects. Other side effects include irritability and nervousness, dizziness, headache, depression, and, rarely, psychosis. Unfortunately, as many as 30 percent of patients taking vigabatrin develop potentially irreversible retinal damage that impairs their field of vision. This was examined in animal studies, where vigabatrin led to a deficiency of taurine, an organic acid that's vital to many organs in the body, including the retina and the brain. When animals were supplemented with taurine, the retinal injury from vigabatrin was not observed. We routinely recommend supplementation with taurine for all children on vigabatrin, and prescribe doses of approximately 10 to 30 mg/kg/d divided in two doses. However, there is no evidence that this is effective in children.

Vigabatrin is available as 500 mg white oval tablets and 0.5 g sachets.

Zonisamide

Zonisamide (Zonegran®) is a sulfonamide drug approved to treat focal seizures. Evidence suggests that it is also effective for generalized absence, myoclonic, and tonic–clonic seizures. It is slowly but completely absorbed over three to six hours and is more than 90 percent metabolized in the liver. Its half-life is 40 to 60 hours and is lower when taken with enzyme-inducing AEDs. It is usually given once daily.

Side effects include drowsiness, dizziness, unsteadiness, decreased appetite/ weight loss, stomach discomfort, irritability, headache, mild cognitive problems, and rash. Kidney stones occur in 1 to 2 percent of patients. Children may experience decreased sweating, which can lead to heat stroke. Zonisamide should be used cautiously by patients taking acetazolamide and topiramate or on the ketogenic diet (which may also cause kidney stones). Patients should drink adequate fluids, especially in hot environments. Zonisamide is available as 25 mg, 50 mg, and 100 mg capsules; there is no liquid, sprinkle, or intravenous form.

THE ROLE OF BENZODIAZEPINES IN TREATING EPILEPSY

Benzodiazepines (clobazam, clonazepam, clorazepate, diazepam, lorazepam) are effective as short-term therapy to help prevent or stop generalized and focal seizures. These drugs can also be effective in long-term management of epilepsy (particularly clobazam). Benzodiazepines are also used to treat anxiety. Tolerance often develops within weeks, however, meaning that the same dose of medication has less effect, whether for epilepsy or anxiety. In adolescents with epilepsy and anxiety, there is some potential for abuse and overuse of benzodiazepines.

If Lucy has more than three tonic seizures when she wakes up, we know she will continue like this for more than 20 minutes—unless we stop them with rectal valium.

Benzodiazepines are very commonly used to stop prolonged or repetitive (cluster) seizures. Intravenous forms are available in the hospital; rectal, buccal (between gum and lip), sublingual (under the tongue), and intranasal benzodiazepines can be used outside the hospital. A child who has a characteristic warning that lasts at least 1 to 15 minutes before seizures may prevent the larger seizure by taking a benzodiazepine when the warning begins.

Benzodiazepines' side effects include tiredness, dizziness, unsteadiness, irritability, hyperactivity, drooling (in children with developmental delays), depression, nausea, and loss of appetite. These drugs have the potential to cause more cognitive problems than most other AEDs. One danger for users of these drugs is the tendency to increase the dose as tolerance develops. Overall, the side effects may outpace any benefits. Moreover, even gradual increases over months or years can lead to personality changes (irritability, depression, or decreased motivation) and cognitive problems (impaired memory) that go unnoticed or are attributed to "epilepsy" or "the person's constitution." This is especially common for children with developmental disabilities, often impairing their cognitive function and quality of life.

For children with epilepsy, seizures may become more frequent or more severe if the benzodiazepine dosage is decreased or the drug is discontinued. The longer a person takes the drug and the higher the dosage, the greater the tolerance and the higher the risk of worsening seizure control with a dose reduction.

Despite these limitations, benzodiazepines are used safely and effectively to treat many children. Clobazam has sustained benefits for children with Lennox–Gastaut, focal, and generalized epilepsies. In fact, it is comparable in side effects and seizure control to first-line AEDs such as carbamazepine for focal epilepsy. For seizures that occur mainly during sleep or shortly after awakening, taking benzodiazepines at bedtime can control the seizures and improve sleep.

Clobazam

Clobazam (Onfi®) has a slightly different chemical-ring structure than the other benzodiazepines, a factor that may reduce tolerance during long-term use. Clobazam is effective in treating focal and generalized seizures but is only approved in the United States for patients who are over age two and have Lennox–Gastaut syndrome. It is also used as an add-on drug in focal epilepsy that has not been controlled with other AEDs. Its half-life is 18 to 36 hours, although an active metabolite of the drug has a half-life of 40 to 70 hours. Side effects include tiredness, unsteadiness, irritability, mild cognitive problems, and insomnia. The drug should not be stopped abruptly, owing to the risk of withdrawal seizures. It is produced as 10 mg and 20 mg tablets, and a 2.5 mg/mL oral suspension.

Clonazepam

Clonazepam (Klonopin®) is used to treat absence and myoclonic seizures, and can help stop seizure clusters. Clonazepam is available as a generic drug and as the brand-name Clonazepam. It comes in the form of 0.5 mg, 1 mg, and 2 mg tablets, as well as 0.25 mg, 0.50 mg, and 1 mg oral disintegrating tablets (ODTs). The ODT form can be used as a rescue medication to treat seizure clusters or prevent recurrent seizures.

Clorazepate

Clorazepate (Tranxene®) is used to treat focal seizures as an add-on therapy. Clorazepate is metabolized into active drugs desmethyldiazepam and oxazepam; these three drugs have half-lives of 11 to 62 hours. Clorazepate is available as scored tablets in 3.75 mg, 7.5 mg, and 15 mg doses; as sustained-release round tablets, it comes in doses of 11.25 mg and 22.5 mg.

Diazepam

Diazepam (Valium®, Diastat®) is used to treat status epilepticus and seizure clusters. It comes in two forms: rectal diazepam (Diastat®), which is given by patients' families and caregivers to treat prolonged or serial seizures; and oral diazepam, which can help prevent seizure clusters, though its relatively slow absorption limits its effectiveness. Absorption of the rectal form is considerably faster, but because diazepam can impair breathing, rectal diazepam should only be given at the recommended dose. If seizures do not diminish after the first rectal dose, a second one should be given only with a doctor's approval.

Diastat® and the Diastat AcuDial are available as preloaded syringes for rectal administration of diazepam in doses between 2.5 mg and 20 mg. Other liquid forms of diazepam may also be given rectally (with a very small syringe).

Lorazepam

Lorazepam (Ativan®) is used to treat seizure clusters and occasionally to treat chronic epilepsy. Lorazepam can be given orally, sublingually (under the tongue), and by intramuscular and intravenous injections. It has a half-life of 7 to 14 hours and, like diazepam, can cause serious breathing impairment, especially when given intravenously at higher doses. Lorazepam should only be used as recommended by a physician. It is available in 0.5 mg, 1 mg, and 2 mg tablets.

Midazolam

Midazolam is a rapidly acting benzodiazepine that is used buccally (between the lip and gum) or intranasally to treat seizure clusters and prolonged seizures. Pediatric studies (using doses of 2.5 to 10 mg of midazolam in patients with active seizures) suggest that it is likely more effective than rectal diazepam and is equal in safety to that drug, but may be more rapid in onset and offset. As with other benzodiazepines, the dosage is based on the child's weight. Doses of midazolam are typically around 0.2 mg/kg for each administration. Note that children who receive daily benzodiazepines such as clobazam, or who receive rescue benzodiazepine medications often (more than twice a week), frequently develop tolerance to these drugs, so a higher dose of midazolam is needed to stop seizures. Some compounding pharmacies will prepare midazolam for intranasal administration as a "rescue" medication for prolonged seizures or seizure clusters. Many parents and children find this more convenient and less embarrassing than rectal rescue medication, and they may also benefit from a more rapid recovery period.

HOW DO YOU KNOW IF THESE DRUGS ARE SAFE TO TAKE FOR A LONG TIME?

Doctors know considerably more about the long-term safety of drugs such as carbamazepine, phenytoin, and valproate than about medications approved after 1995. Although safety screens and monitoring are better now, significant problems can still occur. The relatively high and very serious risk of liver or bone marrow failure associated with felbamate was identified a year after FDA approval. In contrast, the hormonal side effects of valproate were first reported nearly 20 years after FDA approval. And although the increased risk of birth defects with valproate was recognized within a decade of its approval, the neurodevelopmental effects on children whose mothers took valproate during pregnancy were not recognized for nearly three decades.

Doctors cannot state with certainty that no new side effects will be identified after long-term use of new AEDs, but the overall safety profile of the new drugs appears more favorable than those of most older drugs, especially regarding long-term effects. For example, gabapentin, lamotrigine, and levetiracetam do not cause bone loss and none of the new drugs cause the peripheral nerve damage or soft-tissue changes associated with phenytoin or phenobarbital. Additional data has often been reassuring. The risk of bone marrow failure appeared high with carbamazepine after initial introduction, but is actually very rare (about 1 in 50,000). One study found nearly a 1-in-50 risk of life-threatening rash in children treated with lamotrigine, but when started and increased slowly, the risks are actually less than 1 in 10,000. The risks and benefits of any new therapy must be balanced. For example, is a 35 percent reduction in seizure frequency worth the possible additional side effects, inconvenience, and cost of a second drug? For some it is and for some it is not.

INVESTIGATIONAL ANTIEPILEPTIC DRUGS

Many new AEDs are currently in development, and there are usually, at any given time, others that have already been approved outside the United States. These drugs are the "pipeline" of future medical therapy, especially for patients with uncontrolled seizures or who experience disabling side effects from the current drugs. New drugs also have the ability to greatly help patients who "seem fine" on current medications. For example, some of these drugs may come with reduced risk of bone loss, sedation, weight gain, and other side effects.

It comes down to one thing: We need more effective and safer drugs. And yet, new drug development remains difficult and expensive. The fact that many new drugs have already been introduced has decreased the incentive for companies to invest in the next round of AEDs, since the market is more saturated than it's ever been. Mergers have created large pharmaceutical companies that are only interested in creating "billion-dollar blockbuster" drugs, and the epilepsy market is less likely to provide these kinds of drugs than other disorders, such as hypercholesterolemia or hypertension, as these disorders are much more common than epilepsy. Even when new drugs are brought from the lab to the patient—a very expensive and lengthy process—too often these potential drugs work using similar mechanisms of action to existing drugs. Instead, we need drugs with new mechanisms, because patients whose seizures are resistant to current drugs that work on sodium channels may be resistant to new drugs that work on sodium channels. New drugs, new mechanisms, more choice: Developing new AEDs may be critical to helping people whose seizures are resistant to current therapy.

Should I Enroll in a Drug Study?

Patients with uncontrolled seizures or troublesome side effects on available drugs may want to consider trying an experimental drug. People with well controlled epilepsy and few side effects should generally not consider enrolling in an investigational drug trial. Most drug studies are performed at epilepsy centers. The best way of finding out about new drug studies is by calling or writing to comprehensive epilepsy centers near your home (see epilepsy.com or naec-epilepsy. org for a list of centers).

Drug studies are reviewed and approved by an institutional review board. This helps guarantee that the risks and benefits are carefully considered. Before

TABLE 10.3: DRUGS CURRENTLY UNDER INVESTIGATION

Drug	Presumed Mechanism of Action	Potential uses
Brivaracetam	Binds SV2A	Focal and generalized epilepsies
Carisbamate	Unknown (carbamate)	Focal epilepsy
DP-VPA	Unknown (possibly similar to valproic acid)	Generalized and focal epilepsies
Ganaxolone	Activates GABA(A) receptor complex	Focal and generalized epilepsies, infantile spasms, Fragile X syndrome
Safinamide	MAO-B inhibitor, inhibits sodium and calcium channels	Focal and generalized epilepsies
Seletracetam	Binds SV2A	Focal and generalized epilepsies
Stiripentol	Unknown	Dravet syndrome
Talampanel	Noncompetitive AMPA antagonist	Focal and generalized epilepsies
Valrocemide	Unknown (possibly similar to valproic acid)	Generalized and focal epilepsies

a child is enrolled, the study must be fully explained and consent obtained in writing from a competent adult, parent, or legal guardian. The principal investigator in charge of the study and the hospital's patient advocate should be available to answer any questions during the study. A patient who decides not to participate in a study should have no fears that the doctor will be upset or withhold other therapies. Table 10.3 lists drugs that are currently under investigation.

CANNABIS (MARIJUANA)-BASED MEDICATIONS

The use of cannabis-based products to treat children with epilepsy has attracted an enormous amount of media attention, as well as interest from parents whose children's seizures are not controlled by available AEDs. Cannabis, also known as marijuana, is a flowering plant that has been used medicinally for thousands of years, yet scientific data on its effectiveness and safety is limited. More than 500 compounds have been isolated from cannabis plants, and most medical interest centers on the plant's 80 cannabinoid compounds. However, the plant's noncannabinoid compounds may also alter brain function and influence seizure activity. The two most abundant cannabinoids in cannabis are the psychoactive $\Delta 9$-tetrahydrocannabinol (THC) and the nonpsychoactive cannabidiol (CBD). THC produces a "high." This high and THC's antiseizure effects result from the compound binding to CB_1

receptors in the brain. CBD does not produce a high and does not bind to these receptors; it works via other mechanisms. There is evidence from animal studies that both THC and CBD have antiseizure properties. In a minority of animal models of epilepsy, THC can make seizures more likely to occur, whereas CBD has not been shown to make seizures worse in any animal models.

Epilepsy is an approved indication in all states where medical marijuana is legal. Yet the approval of medical marijuana (MMJ) by many state legislatures has created a paradoxical situation in which patients and physicians have access to the drug but lack data from large-scale, well-controlled scientific studies. This is largely because federal agencies limit basic and clinical researchers' access to cannabis products. This inconsistency between state and federal policies has led to an enormous gap between cannabis use and reliable data.

Several challenges exist in determining the safety and effectiveness of MMJ as a treatment for children with epilepsy. Because MMJ includes an array of compounds, it's a challenge to reproduce it in a way that maintains consistent amounts and ratios of its various ingredients. Once an MMJ preparation is reproduced in a consistent manner, controlled trials are still needed to determine if the product is safe and effective.

There are an increasing number of commercial sources of CBD that can be obtained from the Internet or mail order services. The FDA recently tested 18 products that were claimed to contain CBD: seven had no CBD and no product had more than 2.6 percent CBD.

In addition to MMJ approved by state legislatures, trials are now ongoing to study the effect of pure CBD in children with Dravet and Lennox–Gastaut syndrome. The current trials use Epidiolex®, which is derived from cannabis plants, although other trials are being planned using CBD manufactured in a laboratory. These studies have the advantage of examining the effects of a single compound that can be given in precisely determined doses.

IS MEDICAL MARIJUANA (MMJ) SAFE?

Many parents of children with epilepsy have used cannabis for recreational purposes and feel a level of comfort with its safety. Further, Sativex (50 percent THC, 50 percent CBD), a drug sold throughout Europe to treat spasms in patients with multiple sclerosis, has very good safety data. Still, the safety of MMJ in children has not been adequately studied. There is a tendency to believe that substances obtained from nature are safe while those produced by humans, such as pharmaceutical drugs, are dangerous. Time and time again, this has proven not to be true. For example, natural substances such as mushrooms or puffer fish can be lethal in tiny quantities, while overdoses of many pharmaceutical drugs cause no long-term effects. Each drug must be considered individually with attention paid to the fact that side effects often vary by the dose, population (females versus males, children versus adults, etc.), and individual sensitivities. There have been no adequate studies on the safety of MMJ sold in state-approved dispensaries.

IS MEDICAL MARIJUANA EFFECTIVE IN CHILDREN WITH EPILEPSY?

People often fall for the commonsense notion that if a product is used and a dramatic effect follows, the product obviously works. Thus, if a child who has numerous daily seizures and failed on 10 drugs becomes seizure-free after starting on an oil rich in CBD, it seems clear that the MMJ was effective in controlling her episodes. This may well be correct, but there are often other explanations; the history of medicine includes hundreds of examples where a therapy that was the "standard of care" by mainstream physicians or by alternative therapists was studied and found to be ineffective—or worse, harmful. The easy fallback reaction to this is to say, "That was then! I've seen these new cases on TV with my own eyes!" Remember, without studies in which both the doctor and patient/parent are blinded to whether they receive a placebo or active study drug, we never know for sure. *When it comes to medicine, common sense on its own can lead you down the wrong path.* Progress in science often comes by overturning common sense and common knowledge.

Randomized controlled trials are the only way to counteract the many biases that can influence anecdotal observations. These biases include selection of certain patients, the tendency for patients to recall positive responses better than negative ones, the mistake of ignoring negative responses or blaming them on other AEDs, discounting failures as due to not using enough MMJ, the placebo response, and more. This is not an indictment of care outside of the medical mainstream—it applies equally to practices undertaken by pediatric neurologists and epileptologists. Which drug a doctor chooses to treat a child with is often based on opinion and bias, but the approval of that drug by the FDA resulted from a rigorous scientific process. We admit that there are shortcomings to this process. Most AEDs that are approved by the FDA are studied in controlled trials for only three months—far too short for assessing potential long-term side effects or loss of effectiveness. Further, many AEDs are only studied for effectiveness in a subset of the overall epilepsy population (e.g., partial seizures).

Given the desperate needs of children with treatment-resistant epilepsy and the relative safety of CBD in adults, as well as the significant side effects associated with existing AEDs, it does make sense for parents to pursue treatment with MMJ for their children in states where it is legal. But in order for these parents to be able to make more rational decisions and for their doctors to be able to make more rational recommendations, in the not too distant future we need to obtain objective data on specific MMJ products for children with epilepsy. At this time, some MMJ practitioners claim that specific combinations or ratios are most effective. It's true that some epilepsy patients may do best with certain ratios or amounts of CBD and THC. Today, however, there is unfortunately little to no scientific data to support these claims. We desperately need more data about the safety and efficacy of MMJ products used "to treat epilepsy."

INTRAVENOUS GAMMA GLOBULIN

Gamma globulin is a substance composed of antibodies found in human blood. Antibodies are substances that help fight bacteria and viruses. Intravenous gamma globulin (IVIG) is used to bolster the immune system and treat autoimmune disorders. Its use in epilepsy patients, especially children with uncontrolled seizures, remains investigational. Although some children may improve with this therapy, many others do not. The children who improve may do so because in their particular cases an inflammatory process is what caused epilepsy. For example, one boy underwent unsuccessful epilepsy surgery. His brain tissue showed evidence of a prominent inflammation, and subsequent treatment with IVIG reduced his seizures more than 95 percent. In cases of epilepsy where an inflammatory or auto-immune mechanism is strongly suspected or proven, such as antineuronal antibodies, IVIG can be beneficial.

Gamma globulin is given as an intravenous infusion, usually in the hospital or at home under close supervision. During the first infusion, the patient must be watched closely, since an allergic reaction that requires prompt treatment is possible. Additional treatments are typically done every two to six weeks, usually as an outpatient. If a patient is going to benefit from IVIG, that benefit is usually apparent in the first few months; the length of therapy varies.

Many patients ask whether human immunodeficiency virus (HIV, which causes AIDS), hepatitis, or other viruses can be transmitted during IVIG treatments. Because of the careful donor selection and sterilization techniques used in preparing gamma globulin, the risk of viral infection is considered close to zero. IVIG is expensive and supply is limited. Insurance coverage and expense should be considered.

GETTING DRUGS OUTSIDE THE UNITED STATES

As mentioned previously, some investigational drugs and other AEDs (e.g., stiripentol) are only approved to treat epilepsy in other countries. These drugs can be imported legally into the United States with a doctor's prescription, either from foreign pharmacies by direct purchase in the country or by a mailed/faxed prescription. However, regulations and enforcement can change and the Food and Drug Administration may hold drugs at U.S. Customs until the treating physician obtains an Investigational New Drug approval. When the medications pass through customs (carried or mailed/delivery service), it may help to have a note from the doctor documenting the patient's epilepsy, the approval of the drug for epilepsy in another country, and the need for its use in this specific case (e.g., failure of U.S. drugs to control the patient's seizures). The supply may be limited to three months at one time, and it's essential to reorder well in advance, as medicines may occasionally be held up at the border. The drugs are usually delivered directly to a patient's home. New York City's Caligor Pharmacy can obtain some foreign epilepsy drugs, but this is expensive; their phone number is (212) 369-6000.

Insurance usually does not cover the costs of drugs that are not FDA approved. However, letters of appeal from both the patient and neurologist documenting the patient's failure to respond to U.S. medications, and also noting the potential costs of alternative therapies such as surgery, can help in obtaining coverage.

SPECIAL DIETS FOR EPILEPSY

Diet has long been used as a tool for treating and managing disease, and clinicians continue to use diet and nutrition to manage chronic illness. In patients with epilepsy, ketogenic diets (KDs) have proven especially helpful. The classic KD was created in 1921 by doctors who noted that fasting could control seizures in some people. The doctors mimicked this effect by limiting a person's intake of protein and carbohydrates. A high-fat, restricted carbohydrate, adequate protein diet forces the body to shift from using glucose to using fat as its main energy source. When the body does this, substances called ketone bodies are produced. The "ketogenic diet" was named after these ketone bodies.

Although this KD proved beneficial to patients with epilepsy, the diet fell out of use in the 1940s after a greater array of antiepileptic drugs (AEDs) was introduced. Use of the diet was rejuvenated in the 1990s. Since then, less restrictive diets have been developed and shown results in epilepsy patients, and the use of dietary therapies for epilepsy has expanded to include adults. These KDs are sometimes classified as alternative epilepsy therapies, because they're considered alternatives to medications or surgical procedures. However, the KDs' success in controlling epilepsy is well documented, and among all alternative therapies it is the one with the most data supporting its benefits.

Roughly half of children on sustained diet therapy achieve more than 50 percent seizure control and nearly a third have a greater than 90 percent reduction in seizures, with one-sixth achieving freedom from seizures. This high rate of success makes the diet an effective and attractive option. Generally, the KD is considered after a child has tried more than two medications and her seizures remain uncontrolled; however, it can be started sooner.

When successful, the KD and less restrictive epilepsy diets often allow a reduction in doses of AEDs. Occasionally, AEDs can be eliminated.

THE KETOGENIC DIET

To understand epilepsy dietary therapies, first you need to be familiar with how a regular diet works. Our bodies get energy from three major macronutrients: carbohydrates, proteins, and fats (see Table 11.1 for examples of typical

TABLE 11.1: MACRONUTRIENTS: TYPICAL FOOD SOURCES

Carbohydrates	Fats	Proteins
• Starches, grains, breads, cereals, pasta	• Oils	• Meat
• Fruits and fruit juice	• Butters	• Poultry
• Dairy: milk, yogurt, soy milk, ice cream	• Margarines	• Fish/Shellfish
• Vegetables	• Nuts and seeds	• Eggs
• Starchy vegetables (corn, potatoes, peas)	• Heavy cream	• Cheese
• Legumes	• Mayonnaise	
• Snack foods; pretzels, chips, crackers	• Avocado	
• Sweets; cakes, candies, pies, brownies, cookies		
• Sugars; jellies, jams, sweet sauces, honey, agave, syrups		

carbohydrate, fat, and protein sources). A regular American diet is approximately 50 to 55 percent carbohydrate, 30 percent fat, and 15 to 20 percent protein. When on a regular diet, the body breaks down (metabolizes) carbohydrates into glucose (sugar), which is used as its main energy source. The body can also use protein and fat as energy, but prefers glucose when it's available. By increasing the proportions of fat in the diet and reducing the proportions of carbohydrates and often proteins, the epilepsy diets get the body to use fat as its main energy source.

With fewer dietary carbohydrates coming in, glucose availability is limited. To maintain energy balance, the body compensates for this by burning up its small carbohydrate reserve within 24 to 48 hours and switches to fats for energy. If there is insufficient fat, the body turns to protein or muscle for energy, which is less desirable. In the KD, the energy comes from an increase in dietary fat, so muscle mass is maintained, as well as energy balance and weight.

Diet Basics

The KD is always high in fat and features very few carbs and limited protein, but the specifics will vary from child to child.

Because a typical KD meal is very high in fat, calories in the KD are controlled to ensure that enough energy is provided to support growth, but not so much that excessive weight gain results. A child's particular diet is individualized and carefully calculated by a registered dietitian (RD) trained in KD management. The individualized diet will stick to a selected ratio, which sets the proportion of

TABLE 11.2: UNDERSTANDING THE KETOGENIC RATIO

The ratio refers to the sum of the weight of fat: the sum of the weight of carbohydrate + protein in a meal.

For example: In a 4:1 meal, there are 4 g of fat for every .5 g of protein and .5 g of carbohydrate

Therefore, if a meal has **12 g of protein and 4 g of carbohydrate, there should be 64 g of fat to make it a 4:1 ratio**

- 64 g fat: 16 g of protein + carbohydrate (12 g protein + 4 g carbohydrate)
- This is a 4:1 ratio

fat in the diet against the proportion of carbohydrates and proteins. Higher ratios mean more fat, less protein, and less carbohydrate (Table 11.2). Ratios range from 1:1 to 4:1. A 4:1 classic diet is roughly 2 percent carbohydrate, 8 percent protein, and 90 percent fat. The RD determines the diet ratio for a particular patient based on that person's protein requirements, energy requirements, and dietary habits and preferences. Higher ratios are generally used in younger children and lower ratios are used in older or larger children who have higher calorie and protein needs. The patient's diet ratio is upheld at each meal and snack.

Metabolic Characteristics

The diet's abundance of fat paired with lower carbohydrate and protein intake results in the metabolism of fatty acids in the liver. This produces ketone bodies (*beta-hydroxybuterate, acetate,* and *acetoacetate*) and leads to a state of ketosis. These ketones fuel the brain's energy needs.

Science is still trying to pinpoint exactly how the KD controls seizures. Ketosis is one of several metabolic changes brought on by the KD. The effect of ketones on seizure activity remains unclear. No definite correlation has been found between blood ketone levels—which are routinely checked in urine while a child is on the diet and can also be measured in the blood directly—and seizure control. In animal studies, blood and urine ketone levels do not always correlate with brain levels. So, ketones may directly suppress seizure activity, or they may merely be associated with many of the other metabolic changes in the brain that suppress seizures, or both. The diet also lowers the child's blood sugar, suppresses the breakdown of glucose and reduces insulin production, which, in turn, activates several very complex metabolic changes in the body and brain. These, as well as other factors, contribute to the diet's antiseizure effect.

Starting the Diet: Keto Boot Camp

Your doctor may suggest the KD for your child after initial attempts at drug therapy have failed. If not, you may want to bring the subject up to the medical team yourself. If you and the doctor move forward with the diet, the first step is an assessment and examination of your child by a neurologist, to make sure the diet is an appropriate therapy. Next, an RD meets with the entire family to provide counseling, training, and nutrition assessment. Finally, it's time to initiate the diet, something that can be done either at home or in the hospital. At NYU Langone Medical Center, we initiate the diet in the hospital after the patient has met with the neurologist and RD. We do not fast patients before the diet, since studies have found that fasting provides no long-term benefits and leads to more short-term side effects during KD initiation compared to patients who don't fast. To improve the diet's initial tolerability, we introduce it in a step-wise manner over three days while the child is observed on video-EEG and his blood is monitored for metabolic changes and sugar levels. In the hospital, we're able to quickly identify and treat any problems during this first phase. This time also serves as "keto boot camp" for the family: parents are trained in meal preparation, meal assembly, sick-day management, and diet maintenance. The RD extensively reviews and finalizes any education the family needs to successfully maintain the diet at home. After discharge, the RD maintains close contact with the family, frequently updating meal plans and fine-tuning the diet for best results. The child will have blood work done one month after starting the diet and every three to six months thereafter to check for any abnormalities, which can be corrected by modifying the diet or introducing supplements. Frequent follow-up with the RD and the KD team is critical to maximize the effectiveness and safety of this diet.

Lifelong Commitment?

How long will my child remain on the diet if it is a successful treatment? The diet isn't a lifelong commitment, and when to wean off of it is a question that can only be answered by a particular child's KD team, in concert with the patient and family. Generally, after two to three years of successful treatment, the team may try weaning. There is no way to predict whether seizure control will be maintained once the patient is weaned, so the diet is weaned slowly. A child can remain on the diet for more than two years, but the risks and benefits should be discussed with parents and caregivers.

If the Diet Doesn't Work

Like all effective medical therapies, the diet is not successful for everyone. The diet usually works in the first four to eight weeks, if maintained strictly, but in some cases takes longer. We usually ask that the patient and family make at least a three-month commitment, to give the diet its best shot. If the diet has not worked after three months, or if the burden outweighs the benefit in the eyes of the caretaker, we will wean the diet and discontinue it.

Who Is a Candidate?

There are no strict criteria that define who is and who is not a candidate for the KD. The diet should be considered for all children who have failed more than two AEDs and who are safe candidates. Very young children consuming formula or pureed baby foods are ideal candidates and we suggest considering the diet sooner rather than later with these patients. Young children are more compliant and open to new food choices than older children, since all table foods are relatively new to them. Children who are fed through a feeding tube are good candidates for the diet, as only a change in their formula is required.

There are some patients in whom the KD is contraindicated (Table 11.3) and some epilepsy syndromes and conditions for which the KD is particularly

TABLE 11.3: CONTRAINDICATIONS TO THE USE OF THE KD	
Absolute Contraindications	Relative Contraindications
Carnitine deficiency (primary)	Inability to maintain adequate nutrition
Carnitine palmitoyltransferase (CPT) I or II deficiency	Surgical focus identified by neuroimaging and video EEG monitoring (because the patient may have better long-term control with surgery)
Carnitine translocase deficiency	Parent or caregiver noncompliance
Beta-oxidation defects • Medium-chain acyl dehydrogenase deficiency (MCAD) • Long-chain acyl dehydrogenase deficiency (LCAD) • Short-chain acyl dehydrogenase deficiency (SCAD) • Long-chain 3-hydroxyacyl-CoA deficiency • Medium-chain 3-hydroxyacyl-CoA deficiency	
Pyruvate carboxylase deficiency	
Porphyria	

Source: Adapted from Recommendations of the International Ketogenic Diet Study Group, E. H. Kossoff et al.

TABLE 11.4: CONDITIONS OR SYNDROMES ASSOCIATED WITH HIGHER RATES OF SUCCESS WITH KD

- Glucose transporter protein 1 (GLUT-1) deficiency
- Pyruvate dehydrogenase deficiency (PDHD)
- Myoclonic-astatic epilepsy (Doose syndrome)
- Tuberous sclerosis complex
- Rett syndrome
- Dravet syndrome (severe myoclonic epilepsy of infancy)
- Infantile spasms
- Children receiving only formula (infants or enterally fed patients)

Source: *Adapted from Recommendations of the International Ketogenic Diet Study Group E. H. Kossoff et al.*

beneficial (Table 11.4) and for whom the KD should be considered earlier in the course of therapy.

Food on the KD

The variety and creativity of the foods available on the KD have improved greatly as the diet's popularity has grown. Despite the very high fat content, dietitians and caregivers have found innovative ways to incorporate and "hide" the fat in appetizing meals. Numerous blogs, cookbooks, parent support groups, and dietitians can help you take advantage of the diverse meals.

Starting the KD does not mean your child has to completely give up all of his favorite foods and flavors. Ketogenic meals can be made to resemble your child's current favorites. While you can't go to the local pizzeria, you can make a keto pizza at home and season it with pepperoni, sausage, or many other items. Your dietitian will guide you toward creating innovative meals based on your child's dietary preferences and restrictions. The diet can work even for children with food allergies, families with cultural or religious dietary restrictions, and selective eaters. Here is an example of a popular keto meal:

Chocolate Almond Peanut Butter Smoothie

    4:1 ratio

    400 calories, 40 grams fat, 6 grams protein, 4 grams carbohydrate

Ingredients

    20 grams 40 percent heavy cream

    2 grams unsweetened cocoa powder

    18 grams natural peanut butter

    240 grams unsweetened almond milk

    20 grams walnut oil

Directions:
    Weigh all ingredients on a gram scale. Mix together and place in a blender with a small amount of ice. Blend until smooth. Add stevia to sweeten as desired.

Maintaining the KD at School

How a child will follow the KD's strict regimen while at school is a concern for many parents, especially since some children with epilepsy already feel "different." Your dietitian, the school's guidance counselor, and other parents can help you and your child maintain the diet with as little effect on your child's school and social life as possible. Ketogenic meals can be made to look like a typical school lunch. Your dietitian and doctor can help school personnel understand the KD. Birthdays, parties, and snack times can all be coordinated with your child's teacher. For example, if it's another student's birthday and that child is bringing cupcakes for the class, keto parents often make a keto cupcake that looks similar.

Challenges

The diet is a commitment and, although food can be made to resemble old favorites, the diet is a significant lifestyle change. To work, the patient and family must be fully committed to implementing and maintaining it. All meals and snacks must be carefully calculated by the RD and weighed on a gram scale in exact portion sizes by the caregiver. The portions are smaller than typical meals because they are calorie dense (fat has more calories per gram than carbohydrate or protein). Most of the burden falls on the caregiver to prepare meals. Most recipes use homemade products and whole foods, avoiding convenience and store-bought products. This makes prep work and meal assembly time consuming, which can be lessened by preparing multiple meals at once and freezing or safely storing.

Side Effects

The KD comes with potential but usually preventable side effects. The neurological evaluation, blood, and urine tests your child undergoes before starting the diet can identify metabolic conditions for which the KD is contraindicated.

Side Effects When the Diet Is Initiated

Side effects are most common when the diet is initiated, which is why many centers admit patients for this. Hypoglycemia (low blood sugar) and acidosis (blood becoming more acidic) are the main problems to watch for. During the first few days of the KD, blood sugar can drop very low. The medical team will monitor your child and treat low blood sugar if it occurs. If hypoglycemia becomes a persistent issue during initiation of the KD, calories are increased, providing more energy and usually resolving the hypoglycemia. Unlike hypoglycemia, which often has no noticeable symptoms, acidosis presents as sleepiness or vomiting—accompanied by low bicarbonate, carbon dioxide, and pH levels. Acidosis is more common in children taking certain AEDs and can persist throughout the maintenance stages of the diet. It's normal in all children on the diet for their bicarbonate, carbon dioxide, and pH levels to drop a bit, since the state of ketosis can create an acidic environment. However, if a patient is symptomatic and these levels are dropping too quickly, extra fluids and sometimes a bicarbonate solution is given. If a patient is taking one of the specific AEDs that commonly cause acidosis in conjunction with the diet, the RD and doctors will usually prescribe a buffering agent (such as citrates, baking soda, phosphate, and potassium supplements) to maintain normal bicarbonate and pH levels. Acidosis and hypoglycemia are usually limited to the initiation phase and often resolve without intervention. This is why the KD is initiated to an inpatient, so that the team may monitor and resolve side effects if they occur.

Side Effects During Maintenance

The most common side effect of the KD during its maintenance phase is constipation. This can be avoided by including enough fiber in your child's diet, making sure he gets activity as tolerated, and encouraging liquid intake. If constipation persists, more fiber, more fluids, and certain oils that help promote regular bowel movements are increased. Also, over-the-counter products such as stool softeners (Colace, Senokot), polyethelene glycol (MiraLax), suppositories, and enemas that are "keto-friendly" can alleviate the problem.

There's an increased risk of kidney stones while on the diet: one in 20 children will develop them. The children at highest risk are those who have a family history of kidney stones and those who are taking a carbonic anhydrase inhibitor (zonisamide, topiramate, or acetazolamide). To help avoid kidney stones, we encourage fluids and correct acidosis with a "buffering agent." If there is a family history of kidney stones, tell your dietitian and the keto team so they can take steps to reduce this risk.

Parents of children on the diet are often worried that the high-fat diet will raise cholesterol and lipid levels. Cholesterol and lipid levels are elevated in a third of children on the KD. Often, these elevated cholesterol and triglyceride numbers are temporary. Children with persistent and extremely elevated levels of cholesterol and triglycerides often have a genetic tendency (familial hyperlipidemia) that is aggravated by the diet. In these cases, heart-healthy fats and supplements (carnitine and omega-3s) can help reduce triglycerides and cholesterol, or the diet's fat content can be reduced. Rarely, a child must discontinue the diet due to elevated lipids and cholesterol.

Growth Effects

Growth and weight gain are monitored closely on the KD, and for most, these are normal. Small amounts of weight loss can benefit overweight children. In some cases linear growth (height) slows on the diet, but most children often "catch up" and achieve normal height and weight after the diet is discontinued. Calories and protein can be increased to encourage weight gain and growth while still trying to maintain the same level of seizure control.

More commonly, the diet's restrictions on carbohydrate intake make it nutritionally incomplete and can cause nutritional imbalances. Your child's dietitian will design a supplement regimen to meet your child's nutrition needs. Most children meet their micronutrient needs with a varied diet, a low-carbohydrate multivitamin, and a calcium and vitamin D supplement. Depending on your child's age, he may need additional supplements, such as over-the-counter magnesium, selenium, phosphorus, potassium, and omega-3s. No supplement should be started before speaking with your keto team to make sure it is safe and compatible with the diet. Blood work at the start of the diet, again at one and four months after beginning the diet, and finally at six-month intervals will check for nutritional deficiencies and other abnormalities, ensuring prompt correction if any are found.

Epilepsy affected my life for five years when I finally overcame my hesitation and decided I should do anything to get rid of these seizures. My support system, which included my family (specifically my mom), friends, and community, made the diet possible. Though a lot of attention was put on me for two years, the diet became [the] norm and was worth it because I am now seizure free! All people struggling with epilepsy [should] consider this diet—it has given me my life back. ■ ■ ■

MODIFIED KETOGENIC DIETS

Alternative or modified KDs have been created in response to the challenges and restrictive nature of the KD, including the modified Atkins diet (MAD), the low–glycemic index treatment (LGIT), and the medium-chain triglyceride (MCT) KD. These diets provide more liberty in meal planning, but they still exclude most sweets, grains, breads, and pastas. The alternative diets all strive to mimic the KD's metabolic characteristics by also maintaining ketosis and stabilizing blood sugar. These diets must be implemented under the supervision of an experienced neurologist and dietitian and require medical monitoring.

The Modified Atkins Diet

The MAD (also referred to as a modified KD) is a less restrictive version of the classic KD. Its high-fat, low-carbohydrate, moderate-protein regimen resembles a 1:1 or 2:1 KD and is roughly 60 to 80 percent fat. Its aim is to control seizures with a more palatable and sustainable regimen than the KD.

The MAD can be initiated without fasting or hospital admission. Food on the MAD is not precisely weighed and measured on a gram scale. The diet offers more freedom in the areas of unscheduled meals, protein levels, and calorie intake than the KD. The cornerstone of the MAD is carbohydrate counting. For children, 10 grams of net carbohydrates per day is recommended. Note: Many product labels show only total carbs. Net carbs refers to total carbs less the dietary fiber and must be calculated by subtracting the grams of dietary fiber in a food from the grams of total carbohydrate. Because fiber is not digested, net carbs are most relevant. Ten grams per day is a very small amount of carbohydrate (as a reference point, a one-ounce slice of bread has 15 grams of carbohydrate). Therefore, bread, grains, cereals, sweets, baked goods, and other carbohydrate-rich items are excluded from the diet. Most carbohydrates that a child consumes on the MAD come from dairy, vegetables, fruits, nuts/nut products, and seeds. Fat should make up about 60 to 80 percent of calories on the diet, and therefore butter, mayonnaise, oil, or cream are usually incorporated into each meal.

Data suggests that the MAD and KD yield similar results. The MAD is used in both adult and pediatric patients.

Strict adherence to the diet is critical, especially in the first month. During this time, it's imperative that meals contain the exact amount of carbohydrates and enough fat to sustain ketosis. Urine ketones are checked with ketone strips daily during this first month. Ketones may be high in the beginning and then drop off slightly—a dietitian can help modify the plan to deepen ketosis if necessary.

MAD Specifics: Carbohydrate Counting

Children usually begin the MAD with a limit of 10 grams of net carbohydrate per day. This virtually eliminates most starches, rice, pasta, starchy vegetables, sweets, fruits, and fruit juices. Various methods are available for counting carbohydrates, including books and online applications (reputable Internet-based food databases such as the USDA's are often recommended). Determine which method of counting carbohydrates works best for your family. The RD will teach you how to use the selected program to properly build meal plans that meet the child's calorie and carbohydrate requirements. Foods and meals on the MAD can be made to resemble your child's favorites, including special home-made low-carb bread. Your dietitian's experience, specialized cookbooks, and the Internet can help create innovative and palatable MAD meals.

Initiating the MAD

Since the MAD can be initiated in an outpatient setting—with close follow-up and supervision by the keto team—it can be started right away. Implementation and monitoring of the diet may differ slightly between health care teams. At NYULMC, the dietitian starts with a 60- to 90-minute outpatient counseling session that covers carbohydrate counting, label reading, recipe making, meal planning, and troubleshooting. The family leaves the session with a packet of information to implement the diet and a carbohydrate counter, as well as with recipes, exchange systems, and sample meal plans. The family should prepare its household and obtain the necessary items before beginning the diet. The RD also asks parents to practice making one to two days of meal plans with calculations of carbs, fats, and proteins, so that the meals can be assessed for accuracy. We individualize the MAD, and during the first week we ask for updates so that the diet may be adjusted accordingly.

If a family is willing to take a stricter approach, we encourage a 1:1 or 2:1 hybrid MAD-KD without calorie restriction and uniform meals. With these children, we aim for the nutrient intake of the whole day to resemble a 2:1 or 1:1 diet, and we provide protein, fat, and carbohydrate intake recommendations and counseling on how to achieve these goals at each meal. Some families find this approach easier than just counting carbohydrates, as too much autonomy can cause confusion during meal planning. When there are goals involving all of the food groups, however, these particular parents and families have a more structured idea of what is recommended and find it easier to create meal plans. By focusing on the ratio and specific macronutrient recommendations, we achieve greater ketosis and seizure control without the more severe restrictions of the classic KD.

Don't Forget the Fat

Because there's such a strict limit on carbohydrates in the MAD, those calories must be replaced by an alternate source. Fat is the best way to supplement calories. This urging of the dieter to eat more fat (60–80 percent of calories) is one way that the MAD is unlike the classic Atkins diet but like the KD. Without fat it is difficult for children on the diet to maintain their weight and ketosis. Since the MAD resembles a 1:1 or a 2:1 KD, it involves much less fat than the classic KD.

Vitamin and mineral supplementation is used with the MAD. In addition, all medications are transitioned to carbohydrate-free or low-carbohydrate forms.

The Low Glycemic Index Treatment

The LGIT offers a liberalized alternative to the KD. The LGIT is lower in fat and higher in carbohydrates than both the MAD and the classic KD, and resembles roughly a 1:1 ratio (60 percent fat). The LGIT's regimen is based on a food's glycemic index. *Glycemic index* refers to a food's effect on blood sugar: the lower the glycemic index, the less effect the food has on raising blood sugar. Many factors such as fiber levels, fat content, protein content, and acidity affect a food's glycemic index. Foods with higher fat, protein, acidity, and fiber content usually have low glycemic indexes and cause more gradual elevations in blood sugar as compared to high-glycemic foods.

Low Glycemic Index Treatment Specifics

The LGIT regulates both the quantity and type of carbohydrates. Typically 40 to 60 grams per day of total carbohydrate are recommended, and all of the carbohydrates must be low glycemic (glycemic index of < 50 relative to glucose). The LGIT is individualized to meet each patient's needs, and recommendations for calories, fat, carbohydrates, and protein are provided. Before a child starts the diet, caregivers are educated about carbohydrate counting and about how to use the glycemic index. While on the diet, a child should consume about 60 percent of his calories as fat. Like the MAD, the LGIT does not require weighing and measuring food on a gram scale. Typical household measurements such as cups/ounces/tablespoons can approximate carbohydrate content. The LGIT usually requires vitamin supplementation for balanced nutrition, and blood levels of vitamins are checked at one month and at four months, and then at six-month intervals.

The Medium-Chain Triglycerides Ketogenic Diet

The MCT KD was designed to provide a more palatable and liberal version of the classic diet. The typical fats used on the classic KD (oils, butter, mayonnaise) are mostly long-chain triglycerides that require more complex metabolism than their shorter-chain counterparts, medium-chain triglycerides. MCTs are absorbed more efficiently than long-chain fats and are carried directly into the liver for metabolism. This metabolic difference makes MCTs highly ketogenic, producing more ketones per gram than long-chain fats and reducing the total fat requirement. The 4:1 KD gets 90 percent of its calories from fat; the MCT diet can produce a similar ketosis with only 70 to 75 percent of its energy from fat, allowing more carbohydrate and protein. The MCT diet is often used in children who have low energy needs but high protein requirements. Studies show similar efficacy in seizure control when using the MCT diet compared to the classic KD.

The Medium-Chain Triglycerides Specifics

MCTs can cause diarrhea and abdominal cramps in some children; therefore, the amount of MCT in the diet must be individualized. Typically, children tolerate a balance of 40 to 50 percent of their energy from MCTs and the remaining 25 to 30 percent of their fat from typical long-chain varieties. MCTs should be increased gradually to assure best tolerance. The MCTs in the diet are usually given in a liquid oil form and are calculated into the diet like any other fat. The diet prescription is individualized and the dietitian calculates the amount of MCT oil. The MCT oil is flavorless and can be incorporated easily into foods and recipes. The oil can vaporize and become flammable at a relatively low temperature, so cooking or frying with it at high temperatures is not recommended. Food on this diet is still weighed and measured on a gram scale, and meals are calculated in a ratio to contain specific amounts of carbohydrate, fat, and protein. Because MCT oil is the main fat source, the diet generally has a lower ratio, allowing more carbohydrate and protein. The MCT KD requires vitamin and mineral supplementation.

The diets described here are an effective and attractive treatment for pediatric epilepsy. Although this chapter reviews each diet, entire books have been dedicated to diet therapies for epilepsy; this chapter provides merely a snapshot of what the diets involve. For more information on the KDs, speak with your neurologist or epilepsy dietitian or consult a reputable source listed as follows.

Additional Reading and References

- The Charlie Foundation for Ketogenic Therapies
  www.charliefoundation.org
- Matthew's Friends
  www.matthewsfriends.org
- The Carson Harris Foundation: Parent support group
  www.carsonharrisfoundation.org
- www.epilepsy.com (Epilepsy Foundation)

Recipes and Meal Ideas

- Ketocook
  www.ketocook.com
- Atkins for seizures
  www.atkinsforseizures.com

12 EPILEPSY AND GENERAL NUTRITION

Good nutrition is the foundation for maintaining optimum health, whether you have epilepsy or not. Nutrition gives the body energy, provides a natural defense against illness, and is a cornerstone therapy for managing and treating disease. Maintaining good nutrition involves eating an array of different foods featuring a variety of vitamins and minerals. In aiming for good health, it's important to strive to maintain a healthy weight as well.

While experts agree that eating a variety of foods and avoiding substances that hamper good health are important for proper nutrition, they disagree on which diet offers the best way to do this. Some experts claim sugar is the main culprit in causing disease, and thus advocate for low-glycemic/low-carbohydrate diets. Others say fat, meat, and animal-based diets are responsible for illness. Some argue that calories are to blame, while others claim that specific types of calories are more harmful or more beneficial than others. Evidence is available to support each of these arguments, and simply reading the newspaper on a regular basis will show you that new arguments in this area arise all the time. One thing is for sure: Today's greater availability of calorie-dense food paired with a decrease in physical activity has led to an obesity epidemic in the United States. Yet despite the excess food people are taking in, deficiencies still exist. This is because a healthy weight does not equal optimal nutrition. Proper nutrition requires a balance of micro- and macronutrients, and consumption of all nutrients (vitamins, minerals, and macronutrients such as carbohydrates, fats, and proteins) in moderation. Too much of anything—even a good thing like vitamins—can be injurious.

The "best diet" for an individual depends on her health condition. For example, a person with epilepsy may benefit from a dietary modification such as the ketogenic diet (KD), but the KD will likely not be appropriate for someone with heart disease. As for epilepsy specifically, the only evidence-based nutritional therapies that have been proven successful are KDs referenced in Chapter 11. Certain nutrients may help control seizures, but as of now, there is no proof. Because proper nutrition can improve other disease states, though, it's safe to assume that epilepsy patients could benefit from a healthy body weight and optimal nutrition. These are things, after all, that every person should strive for.

In this chapter, we discuss achieving and maintaining proper nutrition, and also explore other nutrients with potential benefits for epilepsy patients.

MAINTAINING A HEALTHY BODY WEIGHT

The range of body weights that's deemed healthy for your child, as with any person, depends on her height, muscle mass, and general body composition. Body mass index (BMI) is a measurement that takes these factors into account and can be calculated using height and weight (see http://nhlbisupport.com/bmi). Even without doing the calculation, you probably have a sense of whether your child is over- or underweight. If your child is overweight, a healthy weight-loss plan that includes diet and exercise should be implemented. If underweight, you should consult your doctor or dietitian about how to encourage healthy weight gain. Many epilepsy drugs can contribute to weight gain (such as valproic acid, divalproex, gabapentin) or weight loss (topiramate, zonisamide, felbamate). Medical and psychiatric drugs can affect weight as well. If your child is taking any of these drugs, you'll want to keep an eye out for any considerable changes in weight and contact your doctor if the changes are concerning. For children and adolescents who are significantly underweight, consultation with the pediatrician, gastroenterologist, psychologist, or psychiatrist may be helpful.

Whether increasing or decreasing caloric intake to achieve a healthy weight, it's important to maintain a balance of nutrients. The American Academy of Nutrition and Dietetics and MyPlate.gov offer information on how to do this. Table 12.1 reviews the selected dietary messages for consumers based on the 2010 Dietary Guidelines, and is a fine place to start when looking for daily dietary guidance.

TABLE 12.1: RECOMMENDED DIETARY GUIDELINES

Balance Calories
- Enjoy your food, but eat less
- Avoid oversized portions

Foods to Increase
- Make half your plate fruits and vegetables
- Make at least half your grains whole grains

Foods to Reduce
- Compare sodium when selecting foods like soup, bread, and frozen meals, and choose the ones with lower levels of sodium
- Avoid sugary drinks; drink water instead

ONE DIETARY CHANGE TO CONSIDER FOR CHILDREN WITH EPILEPSY: KEEPING AN EYE ON THE GLYCEMIC INDEX

As mentioned already, the KDs are the only therapeutic, proven dietary treatment for epilepsy. But for people with epilepsy who aren't willing to commit to a strict therapeutic diet, a less restrictive diet that's low in both carbohydrates and, notably, refined sugars may be helpful. Many dietitians who counsel epilepsy patients have noticed that even small changes, such as adopting a natural/whole-foods regimen that limits simple and refined sugars, have resulted in improvements in seizures, although no scientific data supports these impressions. These changes—in essence, adopting a healthier, lower-glycemic lifestyle—can be instituted without medical supervision by anyone willing to improve his or her diet.

The key to doing this is keeping an eye on the glycemic index (GI) of all the foods your child eats. Two foods with the same amount of carbohydrates can have different glycemic index numbers, making the way they are digested by the body very different. A low-glycemic diet involves choosing the carbohydrates with favorable (low) glycemic indexes, meaning that these foods are more slowly converted into glucose than foods with higher indexes. Basically, the smaller the GI number, the lower the impact on your blood sugar. Low-GI foods whose carbohydrates are turned into glucose at a slower rate include vegetables and whole grains. Foods with a high glycemic index include refined sugars and bread, which are easier for your body to change into glucose, resulting in a quick increase in blood sugar. A food's GI isn't always easy to discern, since many factors affect a food's GI and many different versions of the GI exist. Sometimes the glycemic index of a food can be found in the product nutrition information; if not, there are several online sources that provide the GIs of common carbohydrates. In looking at these sources, a good key is to remember that an index of 50 or less = Low (good), an index of 50 to 69 = Medium, and an index of 70 or higher = High (bad).

It's worth doing the work to determine the glycemic index of foods your child is eating, since eating lower GI carbohydrates can lead to favorable results not just in terms of weight loss but also a variety of other conditions. Also, because lowering simple sugar intake and transitioning to a lower glycemic diet is healthy for everyone, not just those with epilepsy, this endeavor may be something the whole family can do together. The following step-wise guide can help you and your family begin the journey.

STEP 1: Reduce refined sugars/high-glycemic carbohydrates.
The first step in improving your child's diet and moving her toward a lower-glycemic lifestyle is to eliminate or significantly minimize refined sugars. Refined sugars have a high glycemic index and low fiber content, and thus are absorbed rapidly by the body. This rapid absorption of sugar usually spikes blood sugar and creates a hormonal

cascade that can result in over production of inflammatory hormones and make it easier for the body to store calories (leading to weight gain). By choosing low-glycemic foods that are higher in fiber, you can minimize blood sugar spikes and this hormonal response (see Table 12.2).

STEP 2: Eat fewer processed/packaged foods. The second step to improving your child's diet is to maximize nutrient intake by switching to mostly natural whole foods and eliminating over processed foods. Processed foods are foods that have more than three ingredients (or unrecognizable ingredients). Whole/natural foods usually have the highest concentration of healthy nutrients, and eating them is the best way to make sure the body is getting the vitamins and minerals it needs.

TABLE 12.2: IDENTIFYING, HIGH-GLYCEMIC/REFINED/ SIMPLE SUGARS

- *Simple sugars* is an older term used to describe carbohydrates made of one or two molecules of sugar; *complex carbohydrates* is a term that refers to carbohydrates made of three or more sugar molecules attached together. However, these terms alone do not tell you much about the way the carbohydrates affect your health. The glycemic index (GI) gives you a tool to differentiate between slower-acting "good carbs" and the faster-acting "bad carbs." In order to keep a diet low in the "bad carbs" and higher in the "good carbs," you need to look to food labels and follow these simple rules:
  - Look at a food's ingredients list to distinguish added sugars from naturally occurring sugars. Words like sucrose, glucose, fructose, high-fructose corn syrup, honey, agave syrup, fruit juice concentrates, invert sugar, cane sweetener, maltose, malt syrup, dextrose, and dehydrated cane juice mean there are added sugars in the product. Avoid these if possible.
  - Check total carbohydrates and fiber. The more fiber a product has, usually the lower the GI and the more "complex" it is. Look for foods with more than 2 grams of fiber per serving.
  - Choose whole grains, nuts, legumes, fruits, vegetables without starch, and other foods with a low glycemic index.
  - Decrease high glycemic index foods, like potatoes, white rice, and white bread.
  - As much as possible, avoid eating sugary foods such as candy, cookies, cakes, and sweet drinks.

STEP 3: Choose heart-healthy fats. The third step is to replace unhealthy fats (saturated fats) with healthy fats (unsaturated fats). For years now, dietary fats have been labeled "the bad guy," yet recent research on dietary habits shows that Americans are not overconsuming foods in the fat category. Instead, we're consuming far too many calories in the sugar/carbohydrate category. While it's not recommended to eat a diet high in bad fats (saturated fats), a diet rich in healthy fats that sate hunger pangs can be beneficial for people looking to replace their beloved carbohydrates with something substantial. For people with epilepsy, lowering overall carbohydrate intake and replacing some of those calories with heart-healthy fats is even more beneficial. In fact, heart-healthy fats have earned the nickname "brain food," thanks to their direct role in brain function and the fact that they are an excellent source of energy for the brain— especially in the absence of dietary carbohydrates. *Not all fats are the same*: Some are better than others, and thus reading labels and looking at the saturated versus unsaturated fat balance of a food is important. Fats that are good for the body include those in fish, nuts, vegetable sources, and seeds. Fats that should be limited include those from animal sources such as butter, whole milk, and red meat. Trans fats found in fast food like French fries and in baked goods like cookies should be avoided.

The benefits of a low-glycemic diet include, but are not limited to: weight loss, more consistent energy levels, improved glucose (blood sugar) control, and, in people with epilepsy, sometimes better seizure control. People often report that their energy levels are more even throughout the day when they're following a low-glycemic diet. This is likely due to the absence of sharp blood-sugar spikes and falls. If you think of your blood sugar on a high-glycemic diet as a series of peaks and valleys, after consuming a carbohydrate-dense meal high in simple sugars your blood sugar will increase rapidly to a peak, due to the brisk absorption of sugar. Then, after the meal is digested, your insulin levels (the hormone that helps absorb sugar) will usually become elevated, causing blood sugar to drop to a low valley. Think: peak (blood sugar increase from simple sugars), then valley (blood sugar lows from insulin). The drop from high blood sugar to low blood sugar can cause many people to feel tired. Your blood sugar on a low-glycemic diet is more like a series of rolling hills. You experience less of a blood sugar "spike" (peak) when eating more complex carbohydrates, because these types of carbohydrates are absorbed more slowly than simple sugars. Therefore, you get more of an even blood sugar pattern, which helps maintain more consistent energy levels in some people.

Improving diet is all about balance—too much of a good thing can be bad, and it's important to vary your child's nutrient intake. As a result, aside from recommendations for people on specific therapeutic diets (KDs) to treat epilepsy, we don't recommend cutting out any entire food groups. However, we do recommend re-evaluating your child's nutrient intake and taking careful notice of where she is getting the majority of her calories. Shifting her diet so that she consumes fewer calories from simple sugars, simple carbohydrates, processed foods, and saturated fats, and then having her consume more calories from whole foods such as lean meats, vegetables, fruits, heart-healthy fats, and whole grains, can make a world of difference in the way your child feels.

VITAMINS, MINERALS, AND OTHER NUTRITIONAL SUPPLEMENTS

While most vitamin and mineral supplements pose few major risks, there is no scientific data supporting the claim that vitamins and nutritional supplements can improve seizure control in epilepsy patients, unless a rare deficiency is identified. Many books and websites do assert otherwise, but as far as we are aware, none of the claims that vitamins or supplements lessen seizures are supported by scientific research. The one instance in which vitamins and minerals are proven to improve seizures is in people with rare nutritional deficiencies that cause seizures. Deficiencies in magnesium, calcium, and vitamin B6, for example, can worsen seizures in some patients, and these patients may benefit from supplementation. These deficiencies can only be confirmed through medical assessment, and there is no evidence that supplementation with these vitamins will benefit other children with epilepsy.

If you fear that your child may not be getting all the nutrients she needs from diet alone, in most cases a general multivitamin can provide a safe quantity and a broad range of vitamins and minerals. However, larger "mega-doses" of vitamins and minerals are not well understood and, in some cases, can cause harm.

Some studies have shown that supplements have a beneficial effect on seizures in animals, but less than 1 percent of compounds that show anticonvulsant properties in animals are considered candidates for human treatment, due to efficacy or safety issues. Additional blinded, controlled, and randomized trials must be conducted to answer the questions that remain regarding nutritional supplements, vitamins, and minerals. With all vitamins and nutritional supplements, anecdotal evidence is often based on single cases, small series studies, or uncontrolled human studies. Following, we review the most important findings from the literature to date.

Vitamin B6

Vitamin B6 is an essential vitamin, meaning it cannot be made by the body and must be obtained from diet. It's found mainly in dairy and meat products, as well as fortified cereals and breads. B6 is important for the role it plays in synthesizing neurotransmitters and hormones, balancing electrolyte levels, and lowering homocysteine, a nonprotein amino acid. Elevated homocysteine levels are associated with increased risk of cardiovascular disease. Several rare genetic disorders that cause seizures are related to a deficiency of pyridoxine, a form of B6. These conditions are very rare and are usually diagnosed in the first year by infusing pyridoxine while recording the electroencephalogram (EEG). Genetic testing can confirm the disorder. Pyridoxine deficiencies require lifelong supplementation to prevent seizures. Another way in which a B6 deficiency may be involved in seizures is that several of the body's enzymes require B6 to convert compounds. Deficiency of B6 could reduce the conversion of these compounds, increasing levels of seizure-provoking compounds—and thus increasing seizures. In people without a well-defined deficiency state, though, there is no solid data that B6 supplementation improves seizure control. In addition, although B6 is often used to help counteract the behavioral side effects of the antiepileptic drug (AED) levetiracetam, controlled studies lack the evidence to support this benefit. Very high-dose daily B6 supplements can damage sensory nerves and cause neuropathies, as well as decrease the efficacy of phenobarbital and phenytoin.

Vitamin D

Vitamin D is an antioxidant and key regulator of bone metabolism. AEDs that increase liver metabolism (carbamazepine, phenobarbital, phenytoin, primidone) or otherwise alter liver metabolism (valproic acid, valproate) can increase vitamin D metabolism and lead to osteopenia (mild reduction in bone mineral density) or osteoporosis (modest to severe reduction in bone mineral density associated with increased risk of fracture) in some children. Therefore, combined calcium and vitamin D supplementation (~600 mg of calcium per day and 400–600 IU of vitamin D3 is recommended as part of the daily diet, depending on the child's age) might be warranted for children taking these drugs over several years (~1,000 mg of calcium per day and 800–1,000 IU of vitamin D3 daily if there is evidence of calcium or vitamin D deficiency, respectively).

Antioxidants

Antioxidants are a group of substances that inhibit oxidation reactions in the body and help remove free radicals (compounds that can initiate chain reactions that can disrupt or injure cell components). The brain is particularly vulnerable to injury by free radicals, due to its high metabolic rate. Theoretically, free radicals could lower the seizure threshold due to their effects on the cell (notably in the mitochondrial systems, which can affect neuronal excitability). Although some data suggest that antioxidant levels are depressed in people with epilepsy, the largest and most rigorous study to date found that antioxidant therapy did not improve seizure control. In addition, antioxidants can bind dietary minerals and prevent their absorption in the gut—and some larger-scale studies of elderly subjects showed that antioxidant supplementation was associated with higher rates of cancer and mortality. It is unclear how these studies apply to the general or pediatric populations, but they remind us that too much of a good thing is bad and that everything in moderation is key. Therefore, instead of heading to the vitamin aisle to pick up a bottle of antioxidant supplements, consider instead simply taking a look at your child's diet and trying to increase dietary sources of antioxidants such as colored vegetables and fruits. This is the best way of ensuring that the body gets what it needs.

Minerals

Minerals play a critical role in the functioning of the nervous system. Specific mineral deficiencies can adversely affect health—another reason that balanced nutrition is so important. People with epilepsy seldom need mineral supplementation for seizure control, though changes in diet or mineral supplements may be beneficial if levels of specific minerals are known to be low. Very low levels of sodium, calcium, and magnesium, for example, can alter the electrical activity of brain cells and cause seizures. Low sodium (hyponatremia) can be caused by medications (diuretics, carbamazepine, eslicarbazepine, oxcarbazepine) or by excess water intake, kidney disease, and hormonal imbalances. Low magnesium levels can alter calcium levels, causing them to drop and predisposing a person to seizures. Deficiencies of calcium and magnesium are rare and usually only seen in cases of severe malnutrition or cancer. However, even mild magnesium deficiency can contribute to increased seizure susceptibility. Pilot unblinded studies suggest that magnesium supplements of approximately 450 mg/day can improve seizure control; however, it remains uncertain if magnesium supplements can reduce seizures in specific populations with epilepsy or just in those with slightly low serum magnesium levels. In situations where a child's nutrition is poor (perhaps because of severe GI illness or another health problem) and her magnesium intake may be low or magnesium losses can be high (as in diarrhea), supplements are advisable.

AEDs and also the underlying causes of epilepsy can contribute to mineral deficiencies. One study found that average copper, magnesium, and zinc levels in hair samples were lower in epilepsy patients than in controls. However, serum analysis showed no differences in the average magnesium and zinc levels between patients treated with AEDs and those not. Overall, the research has shown mixed results, and these preliminary studies have to be confirmed before any conclusions or recommendations can be made. As far as we know, AED therapy may not affect trace mineral levels—the condition of epilepsy itself or its underlying causes may account for these differences.

Amino Acids and Other Compounds

Some alternative practitioners recommend nutritional supplements with the amino acids L-taurine and L-tyrosine for people with epilepsy. Taurine is a conditionally essential amino acid derived from cysteine and is involved in cellular functions. Taurine is found in meat, fish, eggs, and dairy products. In animal studies, it's been shown that taurine can help prevent seizures. In humans, there's evidence of a link between taurine and seizures: cerebrospinal fluid taurine levels decline after seizures; levels of taurine in the plasma and urine change after seizures; and associations between increased taurine levels and decreased seizure susceptibility, as well as between decreased taurine levels and more spontaneous seizure activity, have been found. However, only a small fraction of plasma taurine crosses the blood-brain barrier, meaning that dietary supplementation of taurine probably does not significantly alter brain activity. On the whole, dietary taurine's effects on the brain and on epilepsy are uncertain. Small studies have shown that supplementation has variable results.

L-tyrosine is a critical amino acid that forms the building block for several neurotransmitters. Although recommended by some alternative practitioners as a supplement, there is no evidence that tyrosine supplementation reduces seizures.

Carnitine is a compound synthesized from amino acids. Its main function involves transporting long-chain, unbound fatty acids into mitochondria when fat is metabolized into energy. We obtain most of our carnitine needs from meat and dairy, and the body synthesizes the rest. In seizure studies using rodents, carnitine showed neuroprotective properties, but this has not been replicated in humans. Many child neurologists recommend carnitine supplements for children with valproic acid toxicity or who are on long-term valproic acid therapy, since valproic acid inhibits carnitine synthesis and thereby lowers carnitine blood levels. This reduction in available carnitine may increase the production of toxic metabolites of valproic acid, making the drug more toxic to the liver. The supplements are likely not needed, as the carnitine deficiency that results from valproic acid is generally mild, and there's no evidence that the supplementation benefits the average child on valproic acid. Liver toxicity is most common in children under age two years and especially in those under age six months, so most doctors do recommend carnitine supplementation in this group. In general, supplementation with carnitine is safe, and moderate to severe carnitine deficiency can cause problems.

Carnosine is made from the amino acids histidine and beta-alanine. It is most abundant in muscle and brain tissue and has antioxidant properties that modulate levels of zinc and copper. It is unclear if carnosine affects seizure activity in humans or if supplementation alters seizure control. It has antiepileptic efficacy in animal models, but human studies are inconclusive.

Omega-3 Fatty Acids

At the start of this chapter, we talked about the bad reputation that's been undeservedly assigned to fats, as well as the benefits of good fats in a diet. Fats contribute the most calories per gram to a person's diet, yet they also provide compounds important for bodily functions. Polyunsaturated fats, which fit into the healthy/saturated category, are essential and can be taken in via diet or supplements, since the body cannot make them. Two essential (and often promoted in the media) "healthy" polyunsaturated fats are omega-3 and omega-6 fatty acids. The balance of these two fatty acids is very important: Omega-3s have anti-inflammatory properties and omega-6s have pro-inflammatory properties, and the proper balance of the two is associated with lower rates of heart disease. Omega-3s have also shown promise in neuroprotection in animal models. Other animal studies have shown that omega 3s raise the seizure threshold and improve seizure activity. Unfortunately, the seizure protection from omega-3 supplementation in animals was not reproduced in early human trials. That being said, modest supplementation with omega-3 fatty acid may be heart-healthy and is potentially favorable for seizure control. In fact, in 2014 a small, randomized controlled trial suggested that omega-3 fatty acids in the form of fish oil may help decrease the frequency of seizures. In the study, people taking three fish oil capsules a day (1,080 mg of omega-3s) lowered their number of seizures by 33 percent compared to the placebo group. This study is in contrast to previous studies involving higher doses of omega-3s that showed no clear benefits in people with epilepsy. This suggests that taking low doses of fish oil may be a safe, beneficial adjunct therapy in people with treatment-resistant epilepsy. Although this is just a single study, it opens the door for longer, more controlled studies to help us better understand the role of omega-3 fatty acids in seizure protection.

While the idea of nutritional supplementation remains attractive, it's important to remember that none of the supplements covered in this chapter have been definitely shown to improve seizure control, and more studies are needed as a whole in this area. In addition, some supplements may be dangerous or interact with medications; therefore, as with all epilepsy treatments, be sure to discuss any supplements with your physician before using them. If you are seeking a dietary therapy other than the KDs for your child, we recommend following a lower-glycemic, healthy balanced diet, rich in all nutrients and food sources, while making sure to help your child maintain a healthy weight.

References and Further Reading

Blondeau N, Widmann C, Lazdunski M, Heurteaux C. Polyunsaturated fatty acids induce ischemic and epileptic intolerance. *Neurosci*; 2002;109:231–241.

Birdsall TC. Therapeutic applications of taurine. *Altern Med Rev*; 1998;3:128–136.

Collins BW, Goodman HO, Swanton CH, Remy CN. Plasma and urinary taurine in epilepsy. *Clin Chem*; 1988;34:671–675.

Chez MG, Buchanan CP, Komen JL. L-carnosine therapy for intractable epilepsy in childhood: Effect on EEG. *Epilepsia*; 2002;43:65.

DeGiorgio CM, Miller PR, Harper R, Gornbein J, Schrader L, Soss J, Meymandi S. Fish oil (n-3 fatty acids) in drug resistant epilepsy: a randomised placebo-controlled crossover study. *J Neurol Neurosurg Psychiatry*; 2015;86:65–70.

El Idrissi A, Messing J, Scalia J, Trenker E. Prevention of epileptic seizures by taurine. *Adv Exp Med Biol*; 2003;526:515–525.

Freeman JM, Vining EP, Cost S, Singhi P. Does carnitine administration improve the symptoms attributed to anticonvulsant medications?: A double-blinded crossover study. *Pediatrics*; 1994;93(6 Pt 1):893–895.

Gaby AR. Natural approaches to epilepsy. *Alt Med Rev*; 2007;12:9–24.

Isigu H, Matsuoka M, Iryo Y. Protection of the brain by carnitine. *Sangyo Eiseigaku Zashi*; 1995;37:795–802.

Kozan R, Sefil F, Bağirici F. Anticonvulsant effect of carnosine on penicillin-induced epileptiform activity in rats. *Brain Res*; 2008;1239:249–255.

Major P, Greenberg E, Khan A, Thiele EA. Pyridoxine supplementation for the treatment of leviteracetam-induced behavior side effects in children: preliminary results. *Epilepsy Behav*; 2008; 13:557–559.

Oztas B, Kilic S, Dural E, Ispir T. Influence of antioxidants on the blood-brain barrier permeability during epileptic seizures. *J Neurosci Res*; 2001;66:674–678.

Rainesalo S, Keranen T, Palmio J, Peltola J, Oja SS, Saransaari P. Plasma and cerebrospinal fluid amino acids in epileptic patients. *Nerochem Res*; 2004; 29:319–324.

Rabinovitz S, Mostofsky DI, Yehuda S. Anticonvulsant efficiency, behavioral performance, and cortisol levels: A comparison of carbamazapine and a fatty acid compound. *Psychoendocrinology*; 2004;29:113–124.

Schaumburg H, Kaplan J, Windebank A, Vick N, Rasmus S, Pleasure D, Brown MJ. Sensory neuropathy from pyridoxine abuse. A new megavitamin syndrome. *N Engl J Med*; 1983;309:445–448.

Trichopoulou A, Lagiou P. Worldwide patterns of dietary lipids intake and health implications. *Am J Clin Nutr*; 1997;66(4 Suppl):961S–964S.

Wu XH, Ding MP, Zhu-Ge ZB, Zhu YY, Jin CL, Chen Z. Carnosine, a precursor of histidine, ameliorates pentylenetetrazole-induced kindled seizures in rat. *Neurosci Lett*; 2006;400:146–149.

13 | COMPLEMENTARY AND ALTERNATIVE THERAPIES

Complementary and alternative medicine (CAM)—the term we use for the range of practices and therapies that fall outside of standard care—is playing an increasingly large, evolving role in the medical landscape. Traditional approaches such as medications, surgery, and dietary therapy are still considered the ideal, because these approaches are based on evidence and supported by randomized controlled studies. This doesn't mean there's no room for newer approaches. People with epilepsy who continue to experience seizures, side effects, or both while undergoing a traditional medical treatment may find that CAM is an attractive alternative. In this chapter, we explore alternative therapies for children with epilepsy, the evidence or lack of it in support of these therapies, and the risk and benefits of these therapies.

CRANIOSACRAL THERAPY

Craniosacral therapy usually involves gentle physical manipulation of the spine, skull, and cranial sutures, and it is widely practiced, despite limited scientific support for its efficacy.

Since it does not appear to be harmful in any way, however, it may be an attractive option for someone seeking an alternative therapy for epilepsy. Craniosacral therapy is based on the premise that disruptions and interferences in the normal flow of cerebrospinal fluid (the clear fluid found in a person's brain and spine) commonly cause medical symptoms and disorders, and that tapping the skull with the fingertips can free these interferences and restore normal fluid flow. The taps are administered as solid, sharp, nonpainful blows to the head. A minimal amount of force is applied for about 30 to 180 seconds and targets soft tissue structures. The goal is to help the body "self correct" by optimizing the flow of cerebrospinal fluid, opening nerve passages that may be restricted, and aligning bones into their healthy positions. Sessions often last 30 to 60 minutes and are used to treat a variety of neck, skull, head, joint, and other pain syndromes.

Science has yet to prove that craniosacral therapy works. Studies done in the 1970s did not show any proof that cranial bones move or that craniosacral therapy is effective. In addition, there is no real scientific support for the biological plausibility of the therapy and its mechanisms.

STRESS MANAGEMENT, BIOFEEDBACK, AND RELAXATION TECHNIQUES

Some patients with epilepsy report that stress can trigger their seizures. Because stress can alter metabolism, hormones, and chemical activity in the brain and body, it's no surprise that it might also worsen seizures in some people. And while stress is largely thought of as an adult problem, children and adolescents can be under a good deal of stress as well. Think about the pressures children often feel related to schoolwork, friends, sports, and managing their epilepsy. Relaxation techniques that help reduce stress and foster relaxation include breathing exercises, hypnosis, massage, exercise (such as yoga), and biofeedback.

Biofeedback involves learning to control bodily functions that are normally involuntary, such as heart rate. During biofeedback, the person is usually connected to electrical sensors that give information about that person's body. The feedback helps the person focus on making changes, such as breathing to change the heart rate, relaxing certain muscles to achieve pain reduction, and controlling hyperventilation to reduce seizures. Biofeedback rarely makes a person seizure-free, but in helping to reduce stress, it reduces that potential seizure trigger. In addition, biofeedback has become a popular alternative therapy for headaches and migraines—conditions that people with epilepsy often suffer from as well.

Neuro-EEG biofeedback is a specific type of biofeedback that has been used in epilepsy patients, including children. In neuro-EEG feedback, a quantitative electroencephalogram (EEG) is taken to identify abnormal brain rhythms, and then these rhythms are targeted with conditioning to make them more normal and to thereby reduce seizure activity. The sessions last about one hour, one to three times a week for three to 12 months. In 2009, a meta-analysis (analysis involving data from multiple studies) looked at the effectiveness of neuro-biofeedback and showed that 74 percent of patients with medication-resistant epilepsy reported fewer weekly seizures in response to this treatment. None of the studies were controlled trials, so biofeedback should still not be considered a primary treatment for epilepsy, but as there are no known adverse side effects, it may be a good adjunct therapy for some patients. Finding practitioners who are experienced and certified in this technique can be challenging. The Biofeedback Certification Institute of America certifies and oversees practitioner standards; visiting its website can prove helpful in finding an experienced clinician.

Tranquil exercises such as tai chi, yoga, and massage are also wonderful relaxation techniques. Massage is a manual technique in which muscles and connective tissue are manipulated to promote relaxation and alleviate pain. Massage has not been systematically studied in treating people with epilepsy, and no blinded or controlled studies have been conducted to support its use, but those who promote therapeutic massage as an adjunct treatment for epilepsy often note that its relaxation power and ability to reduce stress are helpful. If you decide to go this route, be sure to find a massage therapist who is trained and certified in pediatric massage. Yoga is another relaxation technique that has not been formally studied in treating epilepsy but has been touted for its stress reduction. Some effects of yoga on the EEG and autonomic nervous system have been reported, though no controlled data exists. One study looked at yoga prescribed as a treatment over a six-month period. Patients were divided into three small groups. One group was prescribed yoga, one group performed movements that mimicked yoga, and the third group performed no movements. In the group doing yoga, seizure frequency was reduced by more than 80 percent. No seizure reduction occurred in the other two groups. Stress was also reduced in the yoga group. This study is promising, but these results have yet to be replicated by other researchers. Yoga and massage are generally safe and healthy alternative therapies, but given the lack of hard data, they should not be considered primary treatments for epilepsy. Consider them adjunct therapies that help reduce stress and improve overall well-being. Good news: Yoga classes for children are growing in popularity and are likely offered at your local gym or yoga studio. Seizures during yoga classes should be no more frequent than outside of classes—especially if controlled breathing is learned first to make sure the child doesn't hyperventilate, which can provoke seizures in some children.

EXERCISE

The benefits of aerobic and weight-bearing exercise are well established when it comes to the health of the general public, but less established when it comes to treating epilepsy. As a result, practitioners do not routinely recommend exercise as an adjunct therapy. Many fear that exercise and physical activity may provoke a seizure or cause physical injury—in several studies, exercise-induced seizures have occurred. We can't predict an individual's risk for exercise-induced seizures, what type of exercise will induce a seizure, or how much exercise might induce a seizure. In most cases where seizures are provoked during exercise, it turns out that other factors are involved as well. These factors might include physical and mental tiredness, dehydration, the temperature of the room in which a person is exercising, and the duration and intensity of the exercise. Another common concern among practitioners is hyperventilation, which is known to provoke certain types of seizures. Some clinicians caution their patients to avoid exercise based on this premise. However, a small study in children with absence epilepsy showed that the EEG abnormalities that occur during hyperventilation are not reproduced with exercise. They concluded that children with absence epilepsy should not be discouraged from exercise. More studies are needed to support this hypothesis and to provide recommendations for children with other types of epilepsy. With hyperventilation, blood carbon dioxide goes down, but with exercise, the increase in breathing is because extra carbon dioxide is produced—the increased breathing returns carbon dioxide levels to normal. So hyperventilation and fast breathing with exercise are very different. Other small studies have looked at the effects of exercise in adults with epilepsy. Some found that people who regularly exercise have fewer seizures. One study in particular found that epilepsy patients enrolled in a 15-week exercise program had a significant reduction in seizures compared to their baseline.

We don't know whether the seizure improvement from exercise is directly related to the physical activity or if it's related to the additional physiological benefits gained from exercise. One theory says that exercise works because it improves general brain arousal and increases endorphins (naturally occurring pain relievers); others claim that daily exercise may merely act as a stress reliever. Mood and anxiety disorders are more common in people with epilepsy than they are in the general public. Exercise has been indicated as a treatment for anxiety and depression, so although we lack large controlled studies on the benefits of exercise and epilepsy, it appears that, as a number of small studies have shown, if nothing else, exercise may lead to a welcome improvement in mood and anxiety among epilepsy sufferers.

These aren't the only possible benefits exercise can offer people with epilepsy. Many antiepileptic drugs (AEDs) have the potential to increase a person's risk of osteoporosis and fractures, and weight-bearing exercise is a recommended method for strengthening bones in people with this risk. Exercise can also help with weight management, which is a common problem for people with and without epilepsy.

Until better exercise recommendations are established for people with epilepsy, it's safe to say that if a practitioner has cleared your child for exercise, a mild to moderate program (such as walking, using a stationary bike, and yoga or movement programs) can be beneficial and is often a great adjunct program for improving overall health, well-being, and mood. Mild to moderate exercise rarely induces seizures. As with all activity, any exercise program should be individualized based on your child's particular risk of seizures and injury. For patients with frequent seizures who lose consciousness or motor control, the safest exercise is the one that uses the safest apparatus. For example, a stationary bike rather than a treadmill is considered optimal for someone with impaired balance or who is at risk of losing consciousness. Wearing a helmet and exercising in a padded or carpeted area can also be safer for someone with impaired balance. During vigorous exercise, children with epilepsy should be well rested (not sleep deprived), well hydrated, and not overheated. They should pay attention to their body and not ignore warning signs such as auras, lightheadedness, and extreme fatigue. If seizures are well controlled, any degree and type of exercise is OK, including competitive sports.

SLEEP QUALITY

Getting good-quality sleep is another well-established factor in maintaining physical and mental well-being. Poor or inadequate sleep can cause a number of disturbances during the day, including decreased cognition and memory, mood issues, tiredness, and increased risk of seizures in people with epilepsy. Unfortunately, people with epilepsy tend to have more sleep troubles than those without epilepsy, and this can lead to a frustrating cycle of sleep disruption leading to seizures and vice versa. What causes these sleep issues? The factors can include AEDs, mood disorders, nighttime seizures, and a stressful lifestyle. Sleep disorders such as sleep apnea, insomnia, and periodic limb movements can affect children with epilepsy and can increase the risk of nighttime seizures, which nearly always affect the organization and quality of a person's sleep. Some people don't even realize they are having seizures while they're sleeping; their only clue might be that they feel unusually tired the following day. The sleep disorders listed here are potentially serious medical issues, and they should be evaluated and treated by a physician with the appropriate training and background. In addition, a referral to a sleep center for further evaluation and treatment may also be required to correct these issues. For some people, complementary therapies to improve sleep may be helpful. Consider these tips for helping your child get a good night's sleep:

- Have your child avoid stimulants after noon (coffee, tea, cola, or other beverages containing caffeine; chocolate also contains caffeine and should be avoided later in the day). Also restrict high-sugar items such as juice and sweets just prior to bedtime—they require a lot of insulin to be digested, which can interfere with deep sleep.

- Exercise is helpful in getting good-quality sleep, but avoid having your child do stimulating exercise at night (within five hours of bedtime).

- Get your child into a routine; have him go to sleep around the same time each night and wake up at the same time each morning. If naps are needed, keep them to about an hour per day and before 4:00 p.m.

- Have your child avoid TV, computers, and video games just prior to bedtime.

- Make sure all homework is done early in the night so that it does not interfere with bedtime hours. The stress of schoolwork can interrupt sleep if done too close to bedtime.

- Avoid serving heavy meals just prior to bedtime, though a light snack is OK and may be helpful.

- Try a relaxing activity with your child just before bedtime, such as stretching, reading, or singing quietly.

NEUROBEHAVIORAL APPROACHES

Behavioral techniques are commonly used by people with epilepsy to help stop or control seizures. These techniques involve finding changes in behavior that will inhibit seizure activity and will help the person to avoid situations that might bring on a seizure. The most commonly used behavioral techniques are positive thinking; restraining movements; and stimulation through touch, sound, or visual patterns. When choosing a behavioral approach, the first step is to learn what events or triggers happen before, during, and after your child's seizure—and there are several methods for doing this. Parents interested in learning more about behavioral approaches can refer to Table 13.1, which is a summary of approaches. In reviewing behavioral techniques, these researchers found that most of the listed programs increased a person's knowledge about epilepsy and some even helped improve seizure control, quality of life, acceptance of epilepsy, adherence to medication, mood, and adjustment to seizures.

TABLE 13.1: SUMMARY OF NEUROBEHAVIORAL APPROACHES

Exercise Program	Description	Goals
FAMOSES Created in Germany: www.famoses.de	An educational program for children with epilepsy and their parents. Two parallel sets of lessons are conducted for groups of 6 children and groups of 10 parents. The parent and child modules include orientation, basic facts and causes, diagnosis, prognosis, therapies, and socialization.	Improve parent and child knowledge of epilepsy and help them achieve better understanding of the disease to gain more self-confidence and reduce fears regarding epilepsy.
The Penguin penguinproject.org	Uses cartoon penguins to help children 3–15 years old learn and talk about epilepsy in four 1.5-hour sessions. These sessions include learning what epilepsy is, seizure triggers, safety/first aid, how to talk to others about epilepsy, etc.	Guide children through their symptoms and seizures and show them how to overcome or reduce anxiety and live as normally as possible with family and friends. Explain the causes of their epilepsy and treatment.

(continued)

TABLE 13.1: SUMMARY OF NEUROBEHAVIORAL APPROACHES (*CONTINUED*)

Exercise Program	Description	Goals
SEE theseeprogram.com	Two-day, 16-hour weekend seminar using an information medicine model. Appropriate for children 12 and up. Provides education about the medical aspects of epilepsy, impact on the family, coping skills, vocational adjustment, and social functioning.	Provide psychotherapy for people with epilepsy and their family members using an economically practical delivery system (large-audience intervention typically with 100–300 patients and family members).
FLIP&FLAP See: sciencedirect.com/ science/ article/pii/ S1059131109000776	Three parallel sets of sessions for children older than eight years. Uses age-appropriate training materials including cartoons and manuals. A physician and psychologist present the sessions.	Improve disease knowledge, disease-related emotions, communication, self-responsibility, self-management, social participation, educational security.
Be Seizure Smart cdc.gov/Features/ getseizuresmart	An educational intervention for children and their parents via telephone. A nurse conducts three one-hour sessions plus one group session with several families.	Provide individually tailored interventions for each family member by providing treatment and seizure management information according to the individual's knowledge base, addressing unique concerns and fears, providing emotional support.
CEP See: researchgate.net/ profile/ Peter_Bradley4/ publication/ (continued)	Consists of two parallel sets of four 90-minute sessions for groups of 7–10 children and adults. The children's track is led by two professionals and includes understanding body messages, medications, telling (continued)	For children, the goals are enhancing knowledge, self-esteem, self-care, and social communication skills; promoting the child's responsibility and decreasing parental anxiety. Parental goals are to deal with (continued)

(continued)

TABLE 13.1: SUMMARY OF NEUROBEHAVIORAL APPROACHES (*CONTINUED*)

Exercise Program	Description	Goals
49679940_Care_ delivery_and_self- management_ strategies_for_children _with_epilepsy/links/ 0deec51a622341d96 c000000.pdf	others, coping, and balancing their life. The adult track consists of sharing the experience of having a child with epilepsy, making decisions/problem solving, working as a family system, and coping.	the anger, resentment, and grief associated with the loss of a healthy child and to increase their knowledge about caring for a child with a seizure disorder, with the aim of improving their decision-making skills.
Take Charge of Epilepsy epilepsy.com/ make-difference/ public-awareness/ take-charge-facts	Six one-hour weekly parallel sessions for adolescents and their parents in groups of five. Pyschoeducational techniques are used to teach about adolescent issues, medical aspects and healthy lifestyle/attitudes, positive relationships with peers, family coping, stress management, and skill development.	Improve the quality of life of adolescents with epilepsy.
ACINDES See: ncbi.nlm.nih.gov/ pubmed/10856009	Small-group treatment designed for children with epilepsy and their parents. In separate groups, children and parents learn about the child's condition and learn to identify body signals and early warning signs; recognize the elements of equilibrium and identify triggers; understand treatment, alternatives, and the usefulness of a direct patient-physician relationship; handle specific risk situations (identify risks and learn strategies to handle them including emergency and home treatments); and develop appropriate decision-making strategies.	Train children to assume a leading role in the management of their health, and train parents to learn to be facilitators.

Source: *Adapted from Mittan R. Psychosocial treatment programs in epilepsy: a review. Epilepsy Behav 2009;16:371-380 and Richards A, Reiter JM. Epilepsy: A New Approach. New York, NY: Walker and Co; 1995.*

ACUPUNCTURE

Acupuncture is a technique that involves the insertion of very thin needles through the skin at strategic points throughout the body. Western practitioners feel that this stimulates nerves, muscles, and connective tissue to increase blood flow and boost the activity of a body's natural painkillers. Acupuncture is generally considered painless and safe, as long as a certified and experienced practitioner performs the treatment. A review of the literature dealing with acupuncture as a treatment for epilepsy only turns up one pediatric study. In this study, published in China, boys with epilepsy were randomly assigned one of three treatments: Chinese herbs, Chinese herbs and acupuncture, or medication. The boys in each of three groups experienced a seizure reduction of more than 50 percent, and there was no statistically significant difference in the reduction in any of the groups. As a result, the review concluded that there was no strong evidence for acupuncture as a treatment for epilepsy and that more research should be conducted.

HERBAL REMEDIES

Herbal, or natural, remedies are an extremely popular alternative therapy—nearly 20 percent of all patients who take prescription drugs also take herbal supplements. There's a common misconception that a substance that is "natural," like an herbal supplement, is safe to take. Unlike prescription drugs, though, herbal supplements are not regulated by the FDA (this is because they're classified as dietary supplements, not drugs). Therefore, the safety, effectiveness, preparation, and potency of these substances are not regulated by any governing body. In addition, at present there are no published clinical trials on herbal remedies for the treatment of epilepsy that definitively demonstrate their safety, tolerability, or effectiveness. Although some herbal substances are considered safe, others are considered dangerous for people with epilepsy and can actually cause seizures. In addition, some herbs can interact with AEDs, rendering the AEDs less effective—and this can also cause seizures. Table 13.2 reviews some of the most popular herbs that have been suggested—but not proven—to have beneficial effects on seizure control. Also on the chart are herbs that have many AED interactions or may be harmful and should be avoided. Herbs and their safety have not been studied in children, so always use caution and speak with your health care provider before using herbal supplements.

Many of the complementary therapies that we've discussed in this chapter are safe and can be used as successful adjuncts to traditional medical treatment in people with epilepsy. Remember to always discuss these treatments with your health care practitioner to make sure they are safe to incorporate into your child's medical routine. Given the lack of hard evidence for any of the discussed complementary therapies, they should not be considered as the sole therapy for treating your child's epilepsy and seizures. However, many can be used as safe and beneficial additions to the traditional approaches that have been recommended by your medical team.

TABLE 13.2: POPULAR HERBAL REMEDIES ALLEGED TO HAVE BENEFICIAL EFFECTS ON SEIZURE CONTROL

Herb	Proposed Use/Benefit	Possible Interactions/ Adverse Events	Possible Effects in People with Epilepsy	Potential Risks in People with Epilepsy
Chamomile	Relaxation	Can interact with blood thinners/ vomiting, lethargy	None reported	Can intensify or prolong effects of phenobarbital
Coenzyme Q10	Antioxidant; ameliorates neurodegenerative disorders	Use caution if taking blood thinners	May improve seizures in neurological mitochondrial diseases	None reported
Echinacea	Enhances immune system	Gastrointestinal (GI) upset, hepatotoxicity with prolonged use	None reported	None reported
Ephedra	Weight loss, stimulant	High blood pressure, fast heart rate, seizures	None reported	Associated with increased seizures
Evening primrose	Helps with menopausal symptoms	None reported	Antiseizure reports in animals only	May provoke seizures
Ginger	Helps improve GI symptoms, disease prevention; anti-inflammatory	Can increase bleeding in warfarin users	May have antiepileptic effects	None reported
Ginkgo biloba	Improves cognition, cardiovascular improvements	GI upset; interacts with some medications	Leaves and stems may have seizure reduction benefits	Seeds are toxic and may be pro-convulsive; may increase metabolism of some AEDS (phenytoin, valproic acid, phenobarbital)

(continued)

TABLE 13.2: POPULAR HERBAL REMEDIES ALLEGED TO HAVE BENEFICIAL EFFECTS ON SEIZURE CONTROL (*CONTINUED*)

Herb	Proposed Use/Benefit	Possible Interactions/ Adverse Events	Possible Effects in People with Epilepsy	Potential Risks in People with Epilepsy
Ginseng	Improves depression, anxiety, diabetes, sexual dysfunction in men; stimulant	bleeding; possible liver toxicity	May have anticonvulsive properties	May exacerbate seizures
Glucosamine	Anti-inflammatory	None reported	None reported	None reported
Glutamine	Helps healing after sports/injury; pro-immune system	None reported	None reported	None reported
Goldenseal (*Hydrastis canadensis*)	Anti-inflammatory	Can cause hypernatremia and high blood pressure	None reported	None reported
Melatonin	Helps with insomnia, circadian rhythm abnormalities	Nausea, headaches	May benefit seizure control	None reported
Saw palmetto	Prevents urinary tract infection	GI disturbances, headaches	None reported	None reported
Silymarin (milk thistle)	Anticancer, helps with liver	Headache, nausea	None reported	Can increase metabolism and reduce blood levels of valproate

(continued)

TABLE 13.2: POPULAR HERBAL REMEDIES ALLEGED TO HAVE BENEFICIAL EFFECTS ON SEIZURE CONTROL (*CONTINUED*)

Herb	Proposed Use/Benefit	Possible Interactions/ Adverse Events	Possible Effects in People with Epilepsy	Potential Risks in People with Epilepsy
St. John's wort	Improves depression, pain, and attention deficit hyperactivity disorder	Liver toxicity, visual disturbances, GI upset; interactions with MAOIs, SSRIs, oral contraceptives	Possible benefit	Possibly associated with increased seizures; can lower levels of AEDS (phenobarbital, phenytoin)
Valerian	Helps with anxiety, depression, and epilepsy	GI upset, lethargy	May benefit	Can increase sedation caused by phenobarbital

GI, gastrointestinal; MAOIs, monoamine oxidase inhibitors; SSRIs, selective serotonin reuptake inhibitors.

References and Further Reading

The Biofeedback Certification Institute of America. www.bcia.org/i4a/pages/index.cfm?pageid=1

Devinsky, O, Schachter, SC, Pacia, SV. Alternative Therapies for Epilepsy. Demos, NY, 2012.

Esquivel E, Chaussain M, Plouin P, Ponsot G, Arthuis M. Physical exercise and voluntary hyperventilation in childhood absence epilepsy. *Electroecephalogr Clin Neurophysiol;* 1991;79:127–132.

Eriksen HR, Ellersten B, Gronningsaeter H, Nakken KO, Loyning Y, Urin H. Physical exercise in women with intractable epilepsy. *Epilepsia;*1994;35:1256–1264.

Panjwani U, Gupta HL, Singh SH, et al. Effect of Sahaja yoga practice on stress management in patients of epilepsy. *Indian J Physiol Pharmacol;*1995;39:111–116.

Tan G, Thornby J, Hammond DC, et al. Meta-analysis of EEG biofeedback in treating epilepsy. *Clin EEG Neurosci;*2009;40:173–179.

Xiong X, Zhang G, Huang W, Sun J. Clinical observation of acupuncture and Chinese medicine for treatment of epilepsy in children. *J Tradit Chin Med;*2003;10:62–63.

14 | SURGICAL THERAPY FOR EPILEPSY

Surgery can be an excellent option for some children with uncontrolled seizures, or with seizures that are controlled only by treatments with severe, unacceptable side effects. The surgical therapies discussed in this chapter can help these children enjoy a dramatic reduction in or complete control of seizures, as well as a reduction in the medications they're taking. In some children, both seizures and antiepileptic drugs (AEDs) can be completely eliminated after surgery. However, the benefits of surgery must be carefully weighed against the risks. In this chapter we discuss the decision to opt for surgery, and what the main surgical therapies for epilepsy involve.

WHO IS A CANDIDATE FOR SURGERY?

Most children who are candidates for epilepsy surgery have treatment-resistant focal epilepsy. The definition of treatment-resistant focal epilepsy in a child is very individualized. Each case is different. Even for children with focal epilepsy, surgery should never be the first choice of therapy. A child should be treated with *at least* two single drugs and/or with a combination of two or more drugs before surgery is discussed, and diet therapy should also be considered before looking to surgery (unless there is a clear indication for surgery, such as structural MRI abnormality in the brain). Any medications must be given a full chance to work; that is, the drugs should be gradually increased to the maximally tolerated dose. The decision about how many AEDs to try depends on the individual case. What are chances for success with additional medications versus surgery? How well localized is the seizure focus? How harmful are the seizures and AEDs? A child whose seizures persist despite three or more adequate AED trials is unlikely to achieve complete seizure control with any AED. However, some of these children do become seizure-free over time or respond to another AED or AED combination. So, there's no firm line in deciding which of these children overall should opt for surgery. In children who fail three or more medications and have a well-defined seizure focus in an area of the brain that can be safely removed, the benefits of surgery usually outweigh the risks.

Epilepsy surgery has the highest success rate in children who have localized structural abnormalities such as scar tissue, benign tumors, malformations of brain development, and blood vessel malformations. Removal of these benign tumors and vascular malformations can successfully control the seizures. In some cases, however, especially if the seizures have occurred for years, the area of the brain next to the abnormal tissue is also part of the epilepsy network. Removing only the abnormal tissue seen on the MRI scan may or may not control the seizures. Occasionally, the structural abnormality can turn out to have little to do with the uncontrollable seizures. For example, arachnoid cysts rarely cause treatment-resistant epilepsy. Removing the cyst is unlikely to control such seizures unless the cyst is large and exerts pressure on the brain.

WHEN TO HAVE THE SURGERY

Surgery is often performed on children whose seizures have remained uncontrolled for at least one or two years, though in rare cases it's performed on children who've had seizures for less than six months if the seizures are very frequent and severe. This decision must always take into consideration the overall risks and benefits of brain surgery versus the continued course of uncontrolled seizures and multiple AEDs. A patient with an MRI showing temporal-lobe scar tissue and a video-EEG showing seizures arising from that area is an excellent candidate for early surgery, without waiting one to two years, whereas a child with a normal MRI and a video-EEG that shows a widespread area of seizure onset should not be considered for early surgery. Even in these latter cases, surgery should be considered at some point by the child's treatment team if optimal medical management has not proven to be effective. This is because early childhood is a critical time for brain development, and uncontrolled seizures can have a detrimental effect on the developing brain. Yes, brain surgery is a major procedure and carries potentially significant risks, but continued seizures and high doses of medication can also cause long-lasting effects on a child's intellectual, psychological, and social function.

In the end, timing of the surgery is a very individual choice. Some evidence suggests that the earlier the surgery is performed, the better the outcome. Early surgery can reduce the toll that seizures and medication take over many years or decades. Still, children can have epilepsy surgery after 15 or more years of uncontrolled seizures and become seizure-free. Epilepsy surgery may be a last resort for some, but if the child is a good candidate, surgery should be considered after several AEDs have failed.

FREQUENTLY ASKED QUESTIONS BY PARENTS CONSIDERING SURGERY

The doctor told me the risks of doing surgery. What are the risks of not doing surgery?

Many people fail to consider the consequences of ongoing seizures and high doses of several AEDs. For some children with uncontrolled seizures, epilepsy is a progressive disorder that causes a gradual deterioration of memory, mood, and other functions over time. High doses of AEDs can impair mental and physical health. Uncontrolled epilepsy can be fatal. Among adolescents and adults who are epilepsy surgery candidates, the rate of sudden unexplained death (sudden unexpected death in epilepsy [SUDEP]; see Chapter 8) is more than 5 per 1,000 patient years. This means that over the course of a decade, 5 percent will die from SUDEP. Others die from drowning, prolonged seizures, falls, burns, motor vehicle accidents, and suicide. The risk of death from epilepsy surgery, however, is less than 1 in 1,000. If the child becomes seizure-free after epilepsy surgery, the risk of death is similar to that of the general population.

My doctor recommended surgery. Do I get a second opinion? How do I decide?

The decision of whether or not to have surgery is often difficult. Speaking with other parents who have had to make the same choice is helpful. When you only talk to parents whose names and numbers have been given out by the epilepsy center, there is a risk that these parents have been selected because they've had positive outcomes. Internet chat rooms also suffer from a selection bias: They tend to draw families who've had only very positive or negative experiences, so it is worthwhile to seek several sources of information. An excellent source is the epileptologist and epilepsy surgeon who are treating your child.

If there is doubt about whether or not to go forward, or if you are uncertain about the experience of the team at your epilepsy center, seek the opinion of an epilepsy specialist outside that center. In most cases, the second opinion will make a recommendation very similar to the first. When the opinions disagree, ask each to explain their different approaches and reasons. In many cases, it is simply a different view (conservative versus aggressive) or strategy (one-stage versus two-stage). Often there is no "right" answer, so understanding the issues is critical to making an informed decision. You should not think of this decision in terms of "right" and "wrong" choices, but rather as different approaches with different pros and cons. What is "right" for one patient may not be "right" for another.

Is it worth doing surgery if the chances for seizure freedom are small?

Some epilepsy centers only recommend surgery if there is a very high likelihood that the child will become seizure-free. Others also recommend surgery as a "palliative" procedure—to reduce seizures and medication burdens—when the chances for seizure freedom are small. If the risks of harm are small (for example, less than 2 percent) and the chances of clinically significant benefit are moderate (greater than 50 percent), palliative surgery is worth considering.

If epilepsy can be caused by scar tissue and surgery causes scarring, can the surgery cause epilepsy?

Surgical scars from uncomplicated surgery do not cause intractable epilepsy, since scars from surgery are typically much milder than the injuries that cause seizures. Bottom line: If all of the epilepsy-causing tissue is successfully removed, patients usually become seizure-free. Sometimes all of the epileptogenic tissue cannot be safely removed, and some must be left behind. Even in such circumstances, the doctor may be able to remove enough of the tissue to reduce the epileptic tissue burden and accomplish complete seizure control with medication.

CHOOSING AN EPILEPSY CENTER

Choosing an epilepsy center and surgeon can be a challenge. There are advantages in using the team that has provided the child's ongoing epilepsy care. There are also advantages in opting for a team that has extensive experience in your child's disorder and planned surgery. Again, this is something that varies child by child and doctor by doctor. One should feel very comfortable with the treating team, and not feel pressured about a decision.

WHAT TO EXPECT FROM EPILEPSY SURGERY

Merely the thought of brain surgery evokes fears and questions in most people. Doctors, nurses, psychologists, and other parents can answer your questions about the risks, complications, recovery period, and other details. Epilepsy surgery requires a hospital stay of five days to two weeks or longer. The duration of the stay depends on the procedure. A "single stage" removal of epilepsy tissue is the shortest, while a "two-stage" procedure with invasive electrodes (see "Subdural and Depth Electrodes" section) requires more time. Four to six weeks may pass before your child can resume normal activities.

The procedure varies according to the type of operation (discussed in the following sections). The child is usually under general anesthesia. Occasionally, older children are kept awake while areas controlling vital functions such as language and movement are mapped with mild electrical stimulation.

You'll want to establish realistic expectations before the surgery. Some children are completely free of seizures after surgery, and many others have a marked reduction in the frequency or intensity of seizures. In some cases, seizure control remains unchanged. After surgery, most children who become seizure-free still require AEDs, so it's important keep in mind that the surgery is not a complete cure. Children often continue to take the same medication for 6 to 12 months or longer after surgery. Then, some can reduce medication if there are no postoperative seizures and the electroencephalogram (EEG) shows little or no epilepsy wave activity.

After a postsurgery period of seizure freedom, some children will have seizures again. A new seizure, especially if years have passed after surgery without a single episode, can be a huge disappointment. It can seem as if just when the epilepsy moved into the background of a child's life, it has reappeared. In some cases, breakthrough seizures are caused by medication being reduced, due to the child's seizure freedom. In many cases, these episodes result from missed medications, low AED blood levels caused by diarrhea or vomiting, serious infection, sleep deprivation, excessive alcohol intake in adolescents, or other problems. By avoiding these circumstances, the seizures can remain controlled.

PREOPERATIVE ASSESSMENT

Before surgery, studies are performed to identify the area(s) of the brain from which the seizures arise and to make sure these areas do not overlap with areas critical for functions such as language, memory, and movement. Certain areas of the brain can be removed without any changes in intellect, personality, or mood. The removal of other areas may be associated with slight deterioration or, in some cases, improvement in memory or other functions.

Noninvasive Studies

The preoperative assessment begins with a series of consultations and noninvasive tests. Noninvasive tests do not invade the body or involve surgery and, in general, involve little or no risk. The assessment includes:

- History of the child's risk factors for epilepsy, what occurs during seizures, medication trials, and so on
- Medical and neurological examinations
- EEG recording and video-EEG monitoring to record epilepsy waves between and during seizures
- Neuroimaging with MRI, PET, and SPECT to identify structural (MRI) and functional (PET, SPECT) markers of the seizure focus
- Neuropsychological studies to assess cognitive skills to help identify the seizure focus as well as possible complications of the surgery
- Assessment of the child's emotional well-being and parental social supports, with the aim of identifying issues that should be addressed before and after surgery
- Functional MRIs or magnetoencephalography tests are used in some cases

Invasive Studies

The preoperative assessment may also include tests that "invade" the body. Invasive studies are associated with some risk, which varies dramatically among the different types of tests and procedures.

Subdural and Depth Electrodes

Subdural and depth electrodes are invasive electrodes that record electrical activity directly from the brain and can help precisely localize the seizure focus. The decision to use subdural or depth electrodes depends on noninvasive study results and an intracarotid sodium amobarbital test (see "Intracarotid Sodium Amobarbital Test" section). If everything indicates that there's a single seizure focus located outside vital functional areas, most epilepsy centers proceed without invasive electrodes. If the information is inconsistent or indefinite, or if the focus lies near functional brain areas, invasive electrodes are often used to provide a more exact localization.

With these tests, care must be used to protect the child and electrodes during and after the seizures, often in an intensive care unit. The electrodes may be left in place for days to weeks, depending on the case and how quickly seizures occur.

Subdural electrodes (Figure 14.1) consist of a series of small metal electrodes embedded in plastic and arranged as a thin strip or a large grid. They can directly

FIGURE 14.1: Subdural electrodes implanted in the brain.

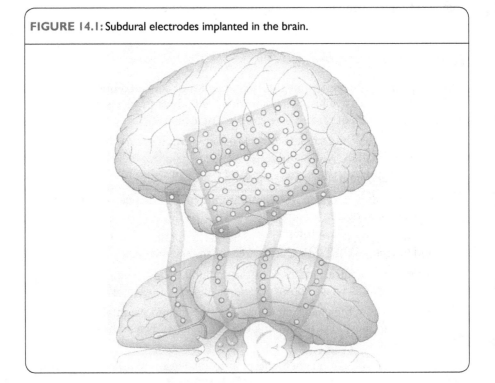

record from large areas of the brain's surface without interference from the scalp and skull. Subdural electrode strips can be inserted through a small "burr hole" in the skull, or a larger grid can be placed after a section of the skull is removed. These electrodes are placed under the *dura mater*, a membrane covering the brain. They do not penetrate the brain. In grid cases, the skull section is replaced or stored frozen in a sterile location, and the electrodes are covered with the dura mater, the scalp, and a surgical dressing. After the testing is completed, the piece of the skull is replaced by re-fusing it to the rest of the skull again. The patient feels moderate pain for several days after electrodes are placed. Pain medicine is given for relief.

Subdural electrodes map brain function by stimulating areas of the brain with mild electrical currents. For example, stimulating the left motor cortex (which controls the right thumb) can cause jerks in this finger. Stimulating language areas in the temporal or frontal lobes can cause a child to suddenly stop speaking. The mapping procedure is almost always painless. The major risks associated with subdural electrodes are infection (which increases during prolonged use, especially after six to eight days), bleeding, and brain swelling.

Depth electrodes (Figure 14.2) are thin, wire-like plastic tubes with metal contact points spread out along their length. Depth electrodes are placed directly into the brain through small burr holes drilled in the skull, and they use computer navigation to localize their placement. Depth electrode recordings, called stereo-EEG, offer the best picture of seizures that arise in areas deep inside the brain, but these

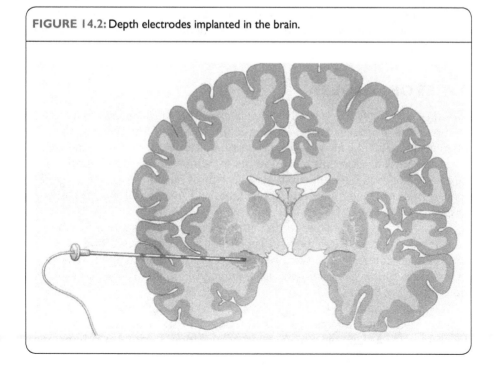

FIGURE 14.2: Depth electrodes implanted in the brain.

recordings cover less of the brain surface than subdural electrodes. Compared to subdural electrodes, depth electrodes are less likely to cause infection or brain swelling, but may have a slightly increased risk of bleeding.

Some epilepsy centers use only subdural, only depth, or both types of electrodes. The decision is often based on the individual case, as well as the expertise and preference of the team.

Intracarotid Sodium Amobarbital Test

The intracarotid sodium amobarbital (Wada) test assesses memory and language functions by putting one hemisphere to sleep with a short-acting anesthetic such as amobarbital, and studying what functions are still working in the other hemisphere. This test is used occasionally in older children and adolescents. To administer the test, a thin plastic tube (catheter) is introduced through an artery in the upper thigh. There is some initial mild discomfort at this point, but the rest of the test is painless. The tube is guided up to the carotid artery in the neck. A small amount of contrast dye is injected and x-rays show blood flow in the brain; some warmth or flashing lights may be momentarily experienced.

Next, the anesthetic is given, which puts almost half of the brain to sleep for several minutes. During this time, language and memory are assessed in the awake cerebral hemisphere. The same procedure may be repeated on the opposite side after 30 to 60 minutes, when the child is fully alert. The risks associated with the amobarbital test are extremely low in children, but stroke is a very rare potential complication.

TYPES OF SURGERY

The most common surgery involves actual removal of the brain area that causes seizures. This *resective surgery* is performed in cases of focal epilepsy. Parents often imagine that the area that causes seizures is tiny—for example, the size of a pea. In almost all cases, the area turns out to be much larger—perhaps the size of golf ball, or even larger in some cases. The most frequent resective surgeries remove parts of the temporal and frontal lobes and are referred to as *frontal* and *temporal lobectomies*.

Less often, surgery is done to disconnect nerve pathways along which seizure impulses spread. These *corpus callosotomy* surgeries involve cutting the large fiber bundles connecting the two hemispheres of the brain without removing brain tissue. *Functional hemispherectomy* surgery disconnects one hemisphere from the rest of the brain.

The least common type of epilepsy surgery is a *multiple subpial transection*. This is used when a person's seizures originate in areas that serve vital functions such as language, movement, or sensation. It can also help people who have Landau–Kleffner syndrome, an acquired language disorder in children in which frequent epilepsy waves affect language areas.

After describing each of these types of surgery in detail, we also look at the surgically implanted vagus nerve stimulator (VNS) and responsive neurostimulation system (RNS), which use electrical stimulation to control seizures.

Temporal Lobectomy

Temporal lobectomy, removal of a portion of the brain's temporal lobe, is the most common and most successful type of epilepsy surgery. In most cases, a modest portion is removed, measuring approximately two and a half inches in length (Figure 14.3). Temporal lobes are important for memory and emotion. In addition, the upper and back part of one temporal lobe is vital for language comprehension. This "language-dominant" temporal lobe is on the left in nearly all right-handed people and most left-handed children. Preoperative tests will assess the potential impact of surgery on memory or language functions. The temporal lobe is a very common location for benign brain tumors in children who have seizures.

The success rate for seizure control after this procedure varies:

- 60 to 70 percent of children will be free of seizures that impair consciousness or cause abnormal movements, but some may experience auras

- 20 to 25 percent of children have a greater than 85 percent reduction of seizures

- 10 to 15 percent of children show no worthwhile improvement

Most children enjoy a marked improvement in seizure control, and thus need less medication after surgery. Approximately 25 percent of those who are seizure-free can eventually come off AEDs.

The risk of a major complication such as a stroke with weakness on the opposite side of the body is less than 1 percent in temporal lobectomy, but this risk varies according to the surgeon. If the surgery extends to the back part of the temporal lobe, there is a risk of loss of vision in the upper quarter of the patient's peripheral vision on the side opposite that of the surgery (Figure 14.4). This impairment rarely affects daily life, and the child is usually completely unaware of it. Less than 1 percent of children will have more frequent or severe seizures after epilepsy surgery.

When surgery is performed on the language-dominant (usually left) side, there is often a mild reduction in memory and in retrieval of infrequently used words. After right-sided (nondominant) temporal lobectomy, memory functions are usually stable or may improve. Children with frequent seizures who achieve complete or nearly complete seizure control and reduced medications after surgery often have better cognitive and mood function. The risk of death from temporal lobectomy is less than 1 in 1,500 patients. The risk of death from uncontrolled seizures is much higher, especially in adolescence and adulthood.

FIGURE 14.3: Brain tissue removed *(shaded areas)* in a standard temporal lobectomy of the left *(top)* or right *(bottom)* hemisphere. (Cross-sectional views, looking from the front, are on the left side of the figure, and side views are on the right.) A smaller amount of tissue is removed from the left hemisphere than from the right hemisphere, because the left temporal lobe contains the area that is vital for language comprehension in most people.

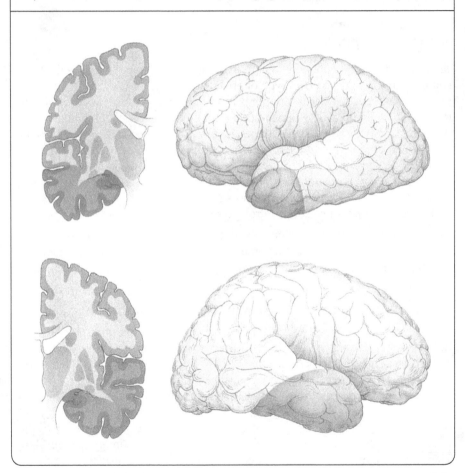

Effects on Personality, Mood, and Behavior

Some parents worry that taking out a piece of their child's brain will result in that child becoming a different person. In fact, long-lasting changes in personality, mood, and overall behavior are rare after temporal lobectomy. Many brain areas perform similar functions. In addition, in children with uncontrolled seizures, epilepsy tissue removed during surgery is often tissue that wasn't functioning properly, and in some cases this tissue was harming other areas ("nociferous" cortex) by "hitting" normal tissue with abnormal electrical activity. Removal of nociferous areas can actually improve a child's cognitive and behavioral function.

FIGURE 14.4: Partial superior quandrantanopsia. The patient's central vision is preserved; only the peripheral vision (to the sides) is affected, and most people are unaware of the problem. In most cases, just a small portion of the shaded region is affected. Patients are usually unaware and unaffected..

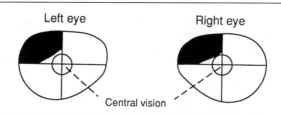

Left eye   Right eye

Central vision

Frontal Lobectomy

After the temporal lobe, the frontal lobe is the second most common site for resective epilepsy surgery. The back part of the frontal lobes (primary motor cortex) controls movement and cannot be removed without causing severe weakness in muscles on the opposite side. In front of the primary motor cortex is the motor association cortex (Figure AA.1). This area links the primary motor cortex with other brain areas. Removal of motor association cortex can cause temporary weakness, but full recovery usually occurs within days to weeks. Other parts of the frontal lobe are involved in personality, executive functions (planning, judgment, reasoning), motivation, and social functions. If the removal of brain tissue is limited to an epilepsy area with a structural abnormality, personality and other functions usually remain intact after frontal lobectomy.

The frontal lobes are large, comprising a third of the brain's cerebral hemisphere (see Figure AA.1). In some cases this makes it challenging to localize the seizure focus.

The success rates for frontal lobectomy are lower than those for temporal lobectomy:

- 45 percent of patients end up free of seizures that impair consciousness or cause abnormal movements

- 30 percent of patients have a greater than 85 percent reduction of seizures

- 25 percent of patients have no improvement or only mild to moderate improvement

The risk of major complications, such as a stroke, is 1 to 2 percent. The risk of behavioral changes is higher than with temporal lobectomy, though behavioral changes associated with frontal lobe impairment are often difficult to measure and define. Changes might affect a patient's personality, motivation, ability to plan and to follow up on a multi-step process or organize actions over time, and social skills. Some children with seizures beginning in the frontal lobes may experience some changes in these behaviors before the surgery. Behavioral improvements can occur after surgery.

Parietal and Occipital Lobectomies

Surgery on the parietal or occipital lobes, located in the back of the brain (see Figure AA.1), is most often performed on patients whose MRI scans reveal a structural abnormality. Invasive electrode recordings may also reveal or confirm that seizures come from one of these areas. The success rate of this surgery in controlling seizures is higher when a structural abnormality is present.

The successes and risks of parietal and occipital lobectomies are similar to those of frontal lobectomy. The risk of muscle weakness is lower, whereas the risk of impairing touch sensation (parietal) or vision (occipital) is greater. On the dominant (usually left) side, the parietal lobe is important for language and skilled motor actions. On the nondominant (usually right) side, the parietal lobe is important for spatial perception and the ability to focus attention toward the left side of space. The occipital lobes are essential for vision. The left occipital lobe receives information about vision in the right half of space, and vice versa.

Corpus Callosotomy

In corpus callosotomy the large fiber bundle (corpus callosum; see Figure AA.1B) that connects the two hemispheres of the brain is cut. Unlike in lobectomy, corpus callosotomy does not involve removing brain tissue. The operation usually entails cutting the front two-thirds of the callosum to reduce seizure frequency and severity. Often a second operation is performed to cut the remaining back third. Corpus callosotomy is most effective for people who have atonic ("drop"), tonic–clonic, and tonic seizures. Seizure frequency is reduced by an average of 70 percent after partial callosotomy and 85 percent after complete callosotomy. Focal seizures often remain unchanged, but may improve or worsen.

The complications associated with corpus callosotomy are greater than those with lobectomy. These complications may involve behavioral, language, and other problems, and may affect function and the person's quality of life. However, serious problems are uncommon and usually temporary. Behavioral problems after callosotomy are most common in people whose language and motor dominance are controlled by different hemispheres; for example, a left-handed child whose left brain controls language and whose right brain controls movement. These potential risks must be weighed against the surgery's possible benefits, such as a reduction in seizure frequency, AED doses, and injuries from falls.

Hemispherectomy

Hemispherectomy originally involved removing half the brain, but now usually involves disconnecting one cerebral hemisphere from the rest of the brain (a procedure called hemispherotomy) and removing only a limited area (Figure 14.5).

This surgery is only considered in children with severe epilepsy whose seizures arise from only one side of the brain in which function is very impaired. Before surgery, the child typically has severe weakness (paralysis) and loss of vision

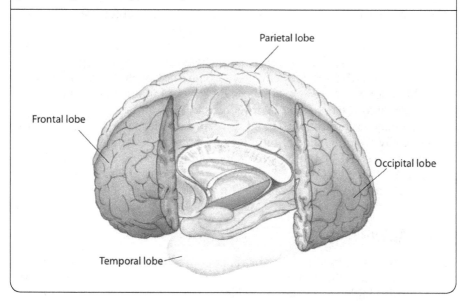

FIGURE 14.5: Outer surface *(side view)* of the left hemisphere, showing the area of brain removed *(light shading)* and the areas of brain disconnected from the opposite hemisphere *(dark shading)* in a hemispherectomy.

Parietal lobe

Frontal lobe

Occipital lobe

Temporal lobe

on the opposite side of the body from where the seizures originate. Therefore, the brain areas that will be disconnected already function poorly, if at all, and the seizures often impair the functions of the intact side. In some cases, when strength and other functions are deteriorating and seizures are coming from one side of the brain (as in Rasmussen's syndrome), hemispherectomy is done despite preserved strength and vision.

When the operation is performed on young children, the opposite hemisphere often helps compensate for the loss. These children will never have movement or normal sensation in the hand, forearm, foot, and leg on the side opposite the operation. However, controlled movements are possible in the upper arm and thigh, thus permitting the child to walk and use the weak upper limb as a "helper." Physical therapy is often needed after surgery.

Hemispherectomy provides complete or nearly complete seizure control in more than 75 percent of cases, including progressive disorders such as Rasmussen's syndrome.

Multiple Subpial Transections

Multiple subpial transection is a surgery that's used to control focal seizures originating in areas of the brain that cannot be safely removed. For example, if the seizures arise from areas that control language or critical motor functions, complete removal would cause permanent language problems or weakness. The operation involves the surgeon making a series of shallow cuts (transections) into the gray matter of the cerebral cortex (Figure 14.6). The surgeon's goal is to selectively interrupt fibers that connect neighboring parts of the brain. The cuts can injure brain cells, but rarely cause long-lasting problems.

In addition to helping reduce or eliminate seizures arising from vital function areas of the brain, multiple subpial transections can improve language function in children with Landau–Kleffner syndrome (see Chapter 3). This procedure can achieve long-term reduction in seizure activity, but it is not as effective as removal or disconnection of the seizure focus.

There may be bleeding at the site of the transection, but transections are generally well tolerated. The procedure may cause mild impairments in the function served by the area operated on, however. The RNS (RNS; see "Responsive Neurostimulation System" section) can also help control seizures from functional areas, without producing any deficits.

Laser Ablation of Seizure Foci

Laser ablation is a surgical option for patients with treatment-resistant epilepsy who have a well-defined seizure focus that shows up as a structural lesion on the MRI (the MRI abnormality must be limited in size for this surgery to be

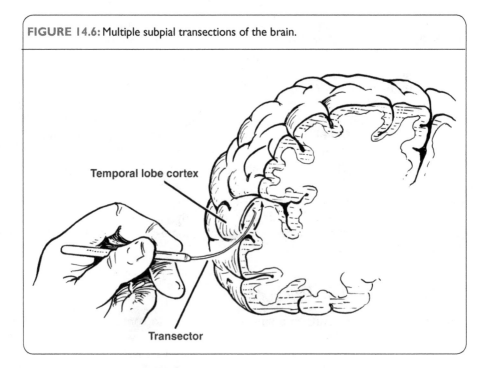

FIGURE 14.6: Multiple subpial transections of the brain.

Temporal lobe cortex

Transector

effective). The main advantage of this treatment is that only a small hole is made in the patient's skull. A laser fiber is guided toward the source of the seizures, using a real-time MRI to confirm the target. The laser heats and destroys the small area of abnormal brain tissue. This procedure has been especially helpful in patients with hypothalamic hamartomas and is also used in other disorders that are still being defined. The risks associated with laser ablation include infection and bleeding as well as injury to neighboring tissue.

Stimulation of the Vagus Nerve

Electrical stimulation of the vagus nerve is another technique for controlling seizures. The vagus nerve is part of the autonomic nervous system—the network that controls involuntary bodily functions such as heart rate. The vagus nerve runs from the brainstem through the neck and into the chest and abdomen. It is a "natural" electrode to the brain, and thus offers a way to influence the brain without opening the skull to do so.

In this procedure, a stimulating device (Figure 14.7) with an approximately five-year battery life is surgically implanted through an incision along the outer side of the chest on the left side. The device is implanted under the skin or muscle for better cosmetic result. A second incision is made horizontally in the patient's lower neck, along a crease of skin, and here the wire from the stimulator is wrapped around the vagus nerve. The child is under general anesthesia during surgery and is usually discharged from the hospital on the

FIGURE 14.7: Vagus nerve stimulator. The generator is implanted under the skin or muscle and the lead wire wraps around the vagus nerve in the neck.

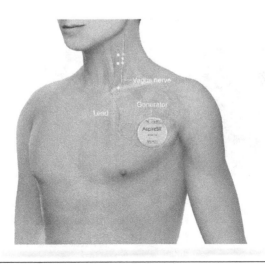

same day. Same day surgery is required to replace the generator when the battery is depleted.

In all patients, the device is programmed (Figure 14.8) to go on for a certain period of time (for example, 7 seconds or 30 seconds) and then to go off for another period (for example, 14 seconds or five minutes). It continuously cycles, intermittently stimulating the vagus nerve throughout the day and night. The programming is independent of when seizures occur. The stimulator can also be easily activated by holding a magnet near the device. The strength of the current delivered after the magnet is activated can be adjusted. For children with warnings (auras) before their seizures, activating the stimulator with the magnet when the warning occurs may help to stop the seizure. However, many patients without auras also show improved seizure control with the VNS. A new Aspire VNS can stimulate the vagus nerve in response to an increase in heart rate for patients whose heart rate increases during more seizures.

Approximately 1 percent of these implants are associated with damage to the nerve that supplies muscles in the voice box, which can result in permanent hoarseness or a change in voice quality. Infection is another potential complication. When the vagus nerve is stimulated, some children experience some change in their voice quality. This is reversible by reducing the stimulation features, but it often diminishes or resolves over weeks or months on its own.

The VNS was approved by the Food and Drug Administration for use in patients with focal epilepsy who are 12 years of age or older. Many centers report success with the device in young children and in patients with generalized

FIGURE 14.8: Programming the device.

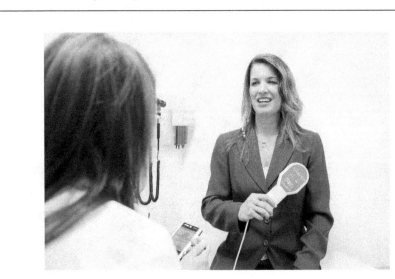

epilepsy and Lennox–Gastaut syndrome. Overall, initial controlled studies reveal that after subtracting the placebo responses, 20 to 25 percent of patients have a 50 percent or greater reduction in seizure frequency after this procedure, another one-third have their seizures reduced by 20 percent to 50 percent, and the remainder do not have worthwhile improvement. Complete seizure control with the VNS is rare.

Responsive Neurostimulation System

This neurostimulator is a programmable, battery-powered device that detects abnormal electrical brain activity and responds by delivering its own short train of electrical pulses to the brain through implanted electrodes. The electrical stimulation aims to normalize brain activity before the patient experiences seizures. The device can be programmed to respond to the specific pattern of a patient's seizure. The neurostimulator is implanted in the skull and connected to two subdural or depth electrodes that are implanted near the patient's seizure focus. The device's battery life is typically four years. Same-day surgery is required to replace the battery when it becomes depleted.

The RNS was approved by the FDA as therapy for patients 18 years of age and older who have treatment-resistant focal seizures that stem from one or two well-localized foci. Although this device has not been approved for use in younger children, it is likely that children over age 12 years—in whom additional growth is predicted to be very slight—may be candidates.

In controlled trials, results of this procedure were similar to those for the VNS. However, many patients in the trial had already failed VNS treatment. After two years of treatment, RNS led to a 50 percent reduction in seizures. Ten percent of the trial patients ended up seizure-free. Complications include bleeding and infection.

EPILEPSY SURGERY DURING THE FIRST THREE YEARS OF LIFE

Infants and young children who have seizures that cannot be controlled with medications are surgical candidates, especially if their MRIs show evidence of abnormalities that are fully or largely restricted to one brain area. This notion, that surgery be considered in even the youngest children, has been an important advance. Studies have shown that uncontrolled seizures are detrimental for the infant brain, that surgery is most often very safe, and that seizure control can also help improve an infant's development. Many children who are candidates for surgery have disorders such as cortical dysplasia or tuberous sclerosis. In some cases, the abnormality is widespread in one entire hemisphere (as in Sturge–Weber syndrome or hemimegalancephaly, in which one side of the brain is abnormally large), and the child's epilepsy is best treated with a hemispherectomy. In most cases, the area is much more limited, and the removal of less tissue can improve or fully control the seizures.

COST OF EPILEPSY SURGERY

Epilepsy surgery is expensive. Because of the complexities involved in the presurgical evaluation, it must be performed at an epilepsy center that has an experienced team. Strategies, philosophies, and costs vary among epilepsy centers, often depending on regional differences and the extent of the presurgical assessment. Invasive electrodes increase cost considerably.

Health insurance covers epilepsy surgery. If the insurance company denies coverage, the patient and the doctor should appeal, as surgery is now a standard medical procedure and considered appropriate, customary care.

III | RAISING A CHILD WITH EPILEPSY

Raising a child with epilepsy often means striking a balance between offering appropriate protection and allowing your child the freedom to learn and grow.

15 | TELLING OTHERS ABOUT EPILEPSY

A lot of people who haven't encountered epilepsy in their own lives have preconceived notions about the disorder—notions based on myths more than on knowledge—and this can make it hard to tell others about your child's diagnosis. Some people, for example, think that children with epilepsy seize nonstop or that the disorder is always unmanageable . . . or always manageable. When you first start telling people close to your family about your child's diagnosis, you'll want to be prepared to correct these kinds of misinformation and answer a lot of questions. A *lot* of questions. You may be asked when and how often your child's seizures happen and whether your child faces a lifetime struggle with the disease. Armed with knowledge, you can help others who are close to your child understand more about epilepsy and how it will affect them.

First, before you tell others about your child's diagnosis of epilepsy, you need to accept it yourself. You need to feel comfortable with the diagnosis and what it means for your family. If your body language or tone conveys fear or discomfort while you're discussing epilepsy, you can ignite the same emotions in the person you're talking to. But if you relate the information to your listeners with confidence and a positive attitude—conveying that this is either a relatively minor problem or one that can be handled with proper precautions and knowledge—they will often respond supportively and will view your child in a more positive light.

TELLING CHILDREN ABOUT EPILEPSY

When other children see Chloe have a seizure, I explain to them, "We all need electricity to use our brains. Sometimes Chloe's brain sends out too much electricity at once and that's what causes her to have a seizure. She is going to be fine and soon everything will be back to normal." ■-■-■

What you tell your own child about epilepsy when you first discuss the diagnosis will depend on the child's age, maturity, and level of understanding. Try to keep the conversation simple, positive, and as truthful as possible. What you're looking for is a balance between providing adequate, accurate information, and making sure that information is easy for your child to understand. Work to avoid new words and ideas, such as medical terms that might overwhelm or frighten your child. You'll also want to avoid trying to protect your child by withholding a basic truth or omitting information that could help her understand the disorder.

Keep in mind that your child may not remember her seizures the way that you do. She might not remember her seizure or seizures at all, in fact, and may only recall waking up to medical care. This can be a frightening and unsure experience, which is why it is important to discuss what happened and to be truthful, yet reassuring.

As for when and whether to talk to your child, in general, children younger than three years do not need to be told anything. After age three, children can usually understand the basic facts about epilepsy if they are explained in simple terms. With young children, a simple explanation of what happened and why mom or dad phoned the doctor is appropriate. If your child is older and more perceptive, you can discuss what a seizure is and what happens in the brain during a seizure. With teenagers, a more in-depth explanation is likely warranted, as many teens may already have misconceptions about epilepsy. Be sure to talk with your child before her first visit to the neurologist or epileptologist to help prepare her and let her know what to expect. Reassure your child that this visit is to help her. If she's old enough, you can help her prepare her own age-appropriate questions for the doctors that you visit.

The way in which you discuss your child's disorder depends not only on your child's age and cognitive abilities, but also on her interest, emotional reaction, and intellectual development. Only you can fully gauge what information your child will be able to understand and handle emotionally, and what information your child will want to know. In addition to a verbal dialogue, a variety of other resources are available to help you explain epilepsy in a child-friendly way (see Table 15.1). These resources range in complexity from simple picture books, to more involved stories that appeal to young readers, to in-depth informational pamphlets that can help your child better understand her diagnosis.

It may take some time for your child to completely digest your discussions about epilepsy and the information you've relayed. In coping with the new diagnosis, your child will likely go through emotional stages similar to those you went through when first hearing the news. Some children fear losing control of their bodies, feel embarrassment about how a seizure looks to others, are scared about feeling different from their peers, and worry about their risk of serious injury or dying from a seizure. Talking with your child and helping her understand the particulars of her epilepsy—as well as how to explain it to friends and classmates—will help her overcome these types of fears.

TABLE 15.1: RESOURCES TO HELP EXPLAIN EPILEPSY TO YOUR CHILD

Books:

- *Mommy, I Feel Funny! A Child's Experience with Epilepsy* by Danielle Rocheford
- *The Great Katie Kate Explains Epilepsy* by M. Maitland DeLand and Jennifer Zivoin
- *Mighty Mike Bounces Back: A Boy's Life with Epilepsy* by Robert Skead
- *Lee, The Rabbit with Epilepsy* by Deborah Moss
- *Is Epilepsy Contagious?* by Julie Devinsky
- *Dotty the Dalmatian Has Epilepsy* by Tim Peters
- *Let's Learn with Teddy about Epilepsy* by Yvonne Zelenka, PhD
- *Taking Seizure Disorders to School: A Story About Epilepsy* by Kim Gosselin

Websites

- www.epilepsy.com/learn/seizures-youth/talking-kids-about-epilepsy
- www.aboutkidshealth.ca/en/resourcecentres/epilepsy/athomeandatschool/copingwith epilepsy/pages/your-child-with-epilepsy.aspx

Depending on your child's age and maturity, consider discussing the following topics:

- What epilepsy is and what it is not (it is not contagious or a psychological illness)
- What types of seizures your child is having
- Tests and procedures that your child may encounter, and how epilepsy is treated and managed
- The ways that living a healthy life helps prevent seizures
- Your child's prognosis, including the fact that the majority of children with epilepsy live full, active, and wonderful lives

More information on coping with the new diagnosis will be covered in the following chapter. In the rest of this chapter, however, we'll discuss the first questions parents often ask after a diagnosis: Who do we want to discuss the diagnosis with, and how?

WHO NEEDS TO KNOW

Relatives

Relatives can be the most supportive people in the world or the most difficult, depending on your family dynamic. As a general rule, close relatives should be informed about your child's epilepsy, especially if they spend significant time with you and your child. You'll want relatives who play an active role in your child's life to be particularly well informed and to learn about basic first aid, so that they can take action if a seizure occurs in their presence. Educating family members can also help allay their fears and dispel myths that might otherwise hurt your child. Urge these relatives not to dwell on the diagnosis or blow it out of proportion, since doing so can cause them to be overprotective and impose unnecessary restrictions that deprive your child of normal experiences. The goal, you should remind them, is for your child to lead the most normal life possible without incurring excess risk.

Some family members may try to give you unsolicited medical or heath advice, and though this advice often comes from a place of caring and love, it can be very irritating. Remember that the decisions related to treatment and management of your child's epilepsy are yours as parents to make, and as parents you should do what you think is best for your child.

School Personnel

Children spend the majority of their weekday hours in school. As a result, their teachers, school nurses, and classmates should be told about the epilepsy diagnosis. The school nurse will be your child's advocate and should also serve as a resource for teachers seeking information. The nurse is most likely the person who will be called if your child has a seizure in school or experiences medication side effects. Make sure to keep the nurse informed about your child's seizure type(s) and features (such as the typical duration of an episode), medications, use of rescue medications (such as rectal diazepam or intranasal midazolam), and potential side effects. The nurse should have your and your child's main doctor's telephone numbers.

Teachers should also be informed about what your child's typical seizure will look like. If your child's teacher isn't already familiar with epilepsy, she should be given a brief education via pamphlets, a video, website, or book describing epilepsy, so that she can learn how to identify a seizure, first aid for seizures, and side effects of medication. Your child's doctor, the school nurse, or a local epilepsy center can help you track down these educational materials. Once a teacher is properly informed, she'll be able to take appropriate action in the event of a seizure and will know how to explain the seizure to your child's classmates. For additional aid in this area, the Epilepsy Foundation's local affiliates provide a free education-based program to schools (see Chapter 22 for more information about the Epilepsy Foundation). The program is called "Project School Alert," and its aim is to help schools become "seizure smart." The program educates teachers and classmates about recognizing different types of seizures, responding to someone having a seizure, providing first aid if needed, giving emotional support to children affected by epilepsy, and how to help others understand. To find out if Project School Alert is available in your region, visit your local Epilepsy Foundation office or go to www. epilepsy.com.

Teachers can also be very helpful in alerting you to behavioral changes that you may not notice at home. These may be behavioral or academic difficulties due to medications or seizures, or psychological and social adjustments to the diagnosis or treatment. It's critical that parents and doctors know about a child's changes in order to make diagnostic decisions (such as whether a drug dose is right) and/or modify therapy.

It's not unusual for children with epilepsy to have more academic difficulties than children without epilepsy, but this very much varies from child to child. Occasionally, a teacher may view a child as having learning problems that aren't there simply because the child has epilepsy. Many children with epilepsy are exceptionally bright students. In some cases where problems occur, they partly result from the psychosocial adjustment to epilepsy rather than a learning disorder. Teachers can help identify any social adjustment issues. That identification can help the parents and teacher manage the difficulties. Teachers are also, ideally, great advocates for children. If necessary, your child's teacher can help the school devise an individual educational program (IEP) to meet your child's needs.

Classmates

The decision to tell young friends about epilepsy is often difficult. Children can be insensitive. In addition, misinformed parents (of children without epilepsy) may fear for their own child's safety and may feel anxious about their child witnessing your child's seizures. Despite these issues, close classmates, friends, and parents of these friends should be told about your child's epilepsy (assuming your child is not yet a teen; for teens, see the next paragraph). The discussion should involve explanations of your child's seizure type, the frequency, how the seizures affect your child, and what to do if a seizure occurs. Most important, your child's friends and their parents need to understand that epilepsy, like asthma, is an episodic problem that affects otherwise normal, healthy children. You want them to know that your child can still take part in most of the activities that she did before she was diagnosed.

For teens and adolescents, who often struggle to fit in even without the added stress of epilepsy, the decision to talk to friends—and which friends to talk to—can be more complicated. Teens should decide on their own if they want to inform friends about their epilepsy. To avoid isolating teens or adolescents, they should always be involved in the decision to reveal their disorder, who to tell, and how to tell them. In general, we favor disclosure, but only with the approval of the teen herself.

Babysitters, Caregivers, and Other Medical Providers

Many parents of young children with epilepsy are scared at the prospect of leaving their children with nonfamily caretakers. And although parents are right in thinking that no one will watch their children as closely as they themselves do, responsible and well-educated babysitters can care for children with epilepsy quite well, giving parents a dose of much-needed freedom. Any babysitters and caregivers who will be alone with your child should be told about epilepsy and about your child's particular seizures before they agree to provide care. They should have a basic knowledge about epilepsy and first aid and, unless they are already familiar with the disorder, should be given the same educational materials you gave your child's school. These caretakers should be reassured that dangerous situations and emergencies are extremely uncommon in most cases, but could arise—hence the need to be prepared. They should know how to identify a seizure, medication dosage, where the medication is stored and how it is given, use of rescue medication, telephone numbers of those to call in an emergency (including your doctor's number), and what to do in an emergency. Making sure that everyone who participates in the direct care of your child is well informed can help minimize your anxiety, your child's anxiety, and the anxiety of these caretakers themselves. In the unlikely event that a caregiver needs to call 911, it is helpful to keep a card with the child's rescue meds, listing basic information the EMS staff might need (date of birth, weight/height, diagnosis, current meds/dosages, parents' cell number and address, and doctor's contact information).

All medical professionals taking care of your child should be informed of the epilepsy diagnosis and should be provided with information about your child's medication doses, If any of these professionals puts your child on a new medication, the professional should review that medication to make sure it won't affect your child's seizure threshold (some drugs make seizures more likely) or interact with any antiepileptic drugs your child may be taking.

INFORMATION IS KEY

Understanding epilepsy and helping your child to understand epilepsy (when age appropriate) so that you can together explain it to friends, teachers, relatives, and classmates is essential in taking back control of your child's life. This enables you to make sure that the people in your life have accurate information about epilepsy and that they understand not just the limits the disorder imposes but also the countless ways that your child is still a typical child. These people should be prepared to respond effectively when necessary and treat your child with informed care.

16 | PARENTING A CHILD WITH EPILEPSY

When your child has a seizure, the physical effects are felt by the child, but the emotional effects spread throughout the family. As a result, parents need to find ways to cope with the fear, confusion, and other feelings that come with seizures and the uncertainties they bring. As with all aspects of epilepsy, how deeply your child's seizures ripple into the family depends on the severity of your child's particular case. If your child's seizures are mild and well controlled, they'll likely not have a major effect on the family. Most children fall into this category and lead lives with few physical or social restrictions. Some, however, even with well-controlled epilepsy, harbor a "dark secret" and live in fear of recurrent seizures. If your child's seizures and antiepileptic drug (AED) side effects cause difficulties, however, all of the members of the family—and their relationships—will be impacted.

Make sure that the disorder and its treatment don't become your family's main focus. Allow your child to continue to be a kid in a household that isn't defined by epilepsy. This can be difficult at first, when the diagnosis is new. Resuming a full life after a devastating diagnosis can be challenging, but it's necessary to provide family structure and normalcy. Once treatment is underway and you have begun to understand and accept the disorder, it's time to actively return to the routines, chores, weekend diversions, and hobbies that filled your life before epilepsy. Think about your child not as a child with epilepsy, but as a child who happens to have seizures.

YOU

Many people worry about everyone but themselves under times of stress. They worry about their child with epilepsy, their other children, spouse, parents, work, and other obligations. In the process of doing everything for everyone, don't forget yourself. A life that was already too busy and overcommitted often becomes unmanageable with an additional stress. Stop and take care of yourself. To be there for your child, you need to be there for yourself. There is nothing wrong with asking for help—from parents, siblings, friends, neighbors, babysitters, and others. And nothing wrong with making sure you have time to enjoy life—see friends, read books, exercise, get a massage, or do nothing.

SIBLINGS

A child with epilepsy draws extra time and attention from her parents, who need to compensate by making special time for their other children. Think of it like this: a child with epilepsy has special needs, but so do her siblings. The book *Views From Our Shoes: Growing Up with a Brother or Sister with Special Needs* by Meyer and Pillo is helpful for young siblings. Spending dedicated time with your other children, no matter how time consuming, will help ward off the natural jealousies that can arise. Recognize the times when extra responsibility is placed on your other children as a result of the epilepsy, as well as when attention is focused largely on the child with epilepsy. You can balance this by making time for the other siblings: extra attention at the dinner table, solo conversations before bed, or special afternoons together at a favorite place or activity. Nothing can replace an open line of communication, involving all members of the family. As the siblings' ages and maturity permit, they should be educated about epilepsy. This education will help alleviate their fears, help them feel a part of what's going on, and help them understand why their parents need to give extra attention to the sibling with epilepsy.

If the diagnosis, communication about the disorder, and integration of treatment into the family's life are handled properly, the impact of epilepsy on your child's siblings can be positive rather than negative. These siblings often grow up to be emotionally stronger, more sympathetic, and more caring. There's no rule about how to discuss epilepsy with your other children. If discussions become difficult or siblings have a hard time coping, you should consider signing them up for sibling workshops or camps. The Epilepsy Foundation runs sibling workshops dubbed "Sibshops" designed to help siblings talk about the specific issues that may arise when a brother or sister seems to get more attention and requires special handling. Allowing siblings to discuss their problems and to connect with others who share their situation can be very beneficial.

SPOUSES

It can come as a shock to discover that your child has epilepsy and possibly other coexisting disorders. The tensions that accompany managing doctors' visits, diagnostic tests, and treatment can strain a marriage. For this reason, divorce may be more common among parents who have children with developmental disabilities than among couples in general. Perhaps more important, bad marriages adversely affect the outcome for a disabled child. You can battle this by recognizing early on in your family's experience with epilepsy that coping with the disorder brings on extra stress, and then—even more critical—making sure that communication with your spouse remains open and honest.

COUNSELING

Despite your best intentions as loving and supportive parents, your children—as well as you and your spouse—may need or benefit from an outside perspective and support as you accept the role epilepsy will play in your life. A counselor can provide that perspective, especially when a child or family member still feels overwhelmed after the facts of the diagnosis have set in or does not know how to feel about the diagnosis. Some people believe that counseling has a stigma attached to it or that getting outside help is viewed as a failure. This couldn't be farther from the truth. Counseling can provide you and your family members with an outlet and perspective on the diagnosis and how to properly cope. Counselors can often help children open up when nothing else is working. Consider school counselors, who may already have background knowledge of your child.

EVERYDAY SAFETY ISSUES

In serious cases of epilepsy, it may seem impossible to resume any sort of "normal" routine as a family, but often it is not. This is another reason that it's especially crucial to develop a comfortable relationship with your child's medical team. They can be an important resource in helping you feel confident as you navigate life with epilepsy. Armed with the recommendations and encouragement of the medical team, you'll need to work hard to set aside your anxieties and concerns about what *could* happen, and make sure that you don't limit your child and hamper her potential based simply on your fears. Most children with epilepsy, especially children with well-controlled seizures, face only slightly greater risks of injury than other children. Even children with more severe, difficult-to-control seizures and other impairments should be encouraged to strive to reach their potential and enjoy a fulfilling day-to-day life.

Plans to ensure your child's safety should be individualized to take into account her particular experience with epilepsy. The type and frequency of the seizures, any medication and its side effects, your child's ability to follow instructions and act responsibly, and the nature and supervision of each particular activity must all be considered. As mentioned in earlier chapters, serious injuries can occur during tonic–clonic, tonic, or atonic seizures. During these seizures, falls may cause bruises or cuts, bone fractures, chipped teeth, sprained joints, or dislocated shoulders. Children with frequent, uncontrolled seizures require special precautions. Common sense should guide all decisions pertaining to your child's safety, aiming toward a goal of both safety and as normal a lifestyle as possible.

STAIR CLIMBING

For most children with epilepsy, stairs are not barriers to getting around. However, seizures that impair motor control or consciousness can cause serious injuries if they occur while the child is on a staircase. This can be frustrating, since stairs—once they're identified as a hazard—seem to be everywhere. If your child has an aura, or warning, before a seizure, she may be able to sit down until the seizure is over and thus avoid being on a staircase at a time when it would be most dangerous. If your child has frequent seizures that cause falling it may be safest for your child to use elevators whenever possible, instead of stairs.

BATHING

Bath time may have to be altered for children with uncontrolled seizures. These children should not bathe in a tub unsupervised. Younger children don't mind this—in fact, bath-time play is an evening highlight for many kids. At older ages, children need privacy. At this point, move your child on to taking showers, which are fine alone. Even then, however, make sure that the bathroom door is never locked. Also, a drain plug that pushes down is dangerous and hot shower taps that can be knocked "on" are also hazardous.

SEIZURE ALERT DOGS

Dogs may be able to sense when a seizure is coming—and then alert the child or their parents by whining or pawing, or in other ways. It's possible that dogs are detecting a subtle change in your child (for instance, an odor or tone of voice) that occurs each time a seizure approaches. Some families believe that having an alert dog, and being aware of these approaching seizures, puts them at ease and allows them to protect their child.

There is no scientific evidence, however, as to whether dogs can really sense an impending seizure. No evidence has been compiled documenting how often the dogs are correct in indicating that a seizure is coming and how often they fail to indicate an approaching seizure.

If you decide that a seizure-alert dog is right for your family and worth the expense (these dogs are costly), you'll want to contact one of the commercial groups that train and sell the animals. The Delta Society (deltasociety.org) and UCB Pharma's canine assistant program (ucb-usa.com/patients/programmes/canine-assistants) can provide helpful information.

BUILDING SELF-ESTEEM IN CHILDREN WITH EPILEPSY

Of all the things that parents can give children, the opportunity to develop self-esteem and self-confidence may be most important. Children must have a strong and positive sense of self to develop, learn, and interact at school, and to grow successfully toward independence. To help your child build healthy self-esteem, parents need to be patient, use educational discipline, provide opportunities for your child to do things independently, and praise her for her initiatives and progress.

As the parent of a child with epilepsy, you need to first maintain your own self-esteem. Having a child with epilepsy can produce a complex mixture of feelings: uncertainty about the future; fears of unpredictable seizures and medication side effects; concerns over stigma that you and your child may face; and all the potential complications of epilepsy, which range from increased risk of attention deficit disorder and depression to sudden death. Most children with epilepsy do extremely well, and knowledge about these risks is often reassuring. For example, rate of sudden death (SUDEP) in children with epilepsy is usually extremely low—for many epilepsies, it's no greater than in the general pediatric population. So before working on your child's self-esteem, you should reflect on your own feelings about your child's disorder. Even very young children can sense and understand their parents' feelings and you want yours to be positive.

This is a good general rule when dealing with your child and epilepsy: emphasize the positive and minimize the negative. Focus on the things that your child can do, and build on those achievements. Negative messages can limit a child's self-esteem and motivation. You need to work hard not to show frustration at what your child cannot do, and you need to refrain from comparing your child negatively with siblings or other children. Talking about "the problem" in front of your child is not good. You can discuss epilepsy in front of your child, but shouldn't do so in a way that casts your child as a problem. The epilepsy should never be the excuse for limiting participation in activities such as school clubs or Scouts unless absolutely necessary. Allowing your child as much freedom as possible, encouraging her to be an active participant in her medical care, and working with her to make and maintain friendships: these will all help strengthen your child's self-esteem.

ENCOURAGE PERSONAL RESPONSIBILITY

Children can understand epilepsy and should be told about the disorder in words they can digest. They need to understand why taking medication on time is important, why tests are done, and why certain activities may have to be restricted. Children usually understand more than adults think they do.

If possible, your child should know the name of her medication, the color of the pills, the dosage, and the medication's schedule. Although it's possible for an attentive parent to do everything in terms of medically caring for a child with epilepsy—allowing the child to become a passive participant in her care—this should be resisted. The earlier that trust and knowledge are given to your child, the sooner the disorder will no longer be a disability to him.

AVOID OVERPROTECTIVENESS

There is a fine line between healthy caution and overprotection. All parents have a strong and natural tendency to want to direct their children's behavior. They want their children to do the things they think are right and avoid things they consider wrong or dangerous. For parents of children with epilepsy, this tendency may become exaggerated, and parents often drift into being overprotective. They may be unaware that their instinct to protect is excessive, or they fiercely defend it. Doing everything for children and restricting their exposure to the usual challenges of childhood takes away the children's independence, slows their social growth, and lowers their self-esteem. They may never learn what it is like to fail or not get what they want. Their peers mature while they remain dependent.

Overprotectiveness can take many forms. In the extreme form, older children may never be told they have epilepsy; they are either told their medications are "vitamins" or simply not told anything. Some children and young adults are overly confined to their houses because of parental fear that they could be injured if they go out. Mild over protectiveness is much more common.

The approach you take to raising your child should include a mix of optimism and realism, allowing them to stretch their boundaries. Children usually survive their parents, and most children with epilepsy will become independent long before their parents are gone. However, many children with severe types of epilepsy and neurological disorders remain dependent and will require some degree of supportive care throughout their lives. If this is the case, be sure to plan ahead of time for your child to eventually live in some type of supportive environment, such as a group home in the community.

ENCOURAGE SOCIAL CONTACTS

The primary skill children pick up during their early childhood is how to socialize. They learn to relate, play, disagree, share, make friendships, and grow with others their same age. Among the greatest costs of overprotection and isolation is how it limits your child's social contacts. No matter how loving you are as a parent, you can never replace the joys and lessons that children bring to each other. Although children can be cruel, you must move beyond the fears of possible problems. Children need other children.

Your child should participate in activities with other children. These activities can range from playgroups and play dates to sports, dancing, singing, or crafts. For older children, independently playing with other children after school and on weekends should be encouraged. Emphasize inclusion, not exclusion. Although you may believe some activities are unsafe for a child with epilepsy, speak with your doctor and child. Special precautions, including closer supervision, can make these activities safer.

Children with epilepsy can feel isolated and sometimes fear rejection by their peers, often unnecessarily. If your child does feel isolated or rejected by her peer group, foster open dialogue with her about her emotions, experiences, and concerns. Asking about her experience opens a door, giving her an opportunity to verbalize her concerns and you a chance to help allay her fears. "How do you feel about having epilepsy?" "How do you think other kids react to you because you have epilepsy?" "Do you understand what the doctor said?" These are all questions that can lead to productive discussions. You want your child to feel comfortable just being a kid.

Children with epilepsy sometimes benefit from meeting, talking, and playing with other children who have epilepsy; it can be enormously comforting for a child to learn that he is not alone. If your area has no groups for children with epilepsy, motivated parents can start one. Camps can also be very rewarding, and Epilepsy.com provides a list of summer camps.

USE EDUCATIONAL DISCIPLINE

Susie has always been impossible. She does what she wants, when she wants. Nothing worked—taking away her favorite toys or foods, sending her up to her room, or raising my voice. We wanted to give up. Then a friend with a child who has cerebral palsy and hyperactivity told me what she thought we were doing wrong. We were inconsistent, often giving in to her tantrums. We reacted to Susie with frustration, never really understanding her needs. It took a lot of hard work. Before Susie could change, we had to change. ■ ■ ■

Some parents of children with epilepsy overindulge them and ignore bad behaviors as a way of making up for the epilepsy or because they fear that sterner punishment will cause more seizures. Although seizures can occasionally be brought on by emotional stress, there is no evidence that seizures are caused by educational discipline. Educational discipline means explaining to your child why the behavior was wrong and withholding something she desires or using the technique of "time out," in which, for example, she must go to the corner of the room and stand quietly for a minute in response to bad behavior. An undisciplined child can face serious problems in learning to socialize in a healthy fashion with other children, to behave and learn at school, and to grow up to be an independent and well-functioning adult. Ultimately, these problems will lead to much greater stress. As early as possible, resist letting your child's disorder get in the way of consistent discipline.

ACCEPTING THE STRESSES OF PARENTHOOD

Very few activities are completely safe for a child with epilepsy—or for a child without epilepsy. Ultimately, whether your child has the disorder or not, she'll face potentially dangerous situations on a regular basis. If you make safety your exclusive concern, you'll unnecessarily limit her activities. Unnecessarily limiting your child emphasizes her disability. This can prevent her from enjoying a full childhood, add to her sense of isolation, or lower her self-esteem. By contrast, don't put your child at unnecessary risk of known danger. Risky activities for your particular child should be avoided or carefully supervised. Just be careful not to put too many limits on your child. All parents stress about the safety and personal development of their children, and it's natural for a parent in a family with epilepsy to stress more than most.

17 | EPILEPSY ISSUES AT DIFFERENT AGES

While parents of children with epilepsy have plenty of immediate worries—"What activities are safe for my child?" "Will my child's new treatment provoke any side effects?"—it's not uncommon to worry about your child's future as well. You may be wondering if your child will outgrow epilepsy, be able to take part in the usual activities of childhood, or enjoy a typical adolescence. The outlook for your child depends on the seizure types, as well as any coexisting disorders and the cause underlying his neurological problems. You can ensure that your child has the best prognosis possible by working with your pediatrician and neurologist to monitor his developmental milestones. The earlier a child who exhibits some delays is enrolled in therapies, the more likely it is that he will improve and progress.

EARLY CHILDHOOD

With young children, be especially alert to issues of self-esteem (which is touched on Chapter 16). As a child's self-image and self-esteem are beginning to develop, they will be influenced by how you view your child and his epilepsy. Children understand and absorb much more than they can express. The fears of their parents, relatives, and caretakers can be imprinted on them. Project positive emotions. Be honest. Especially as your child gets older, accurate and honest information is important, as is trying to include your child in discussions regarding the epilepsy and any potential treatment. Age-appropriate discussions about epilepsy and the reason your child is taking medication, for example, can help him accept his diagnosis. These honest discussions should be geared toward a hopeful tone and away from fear.

ADOLESCENCE

For most children, the passage from childhood to adulthood involves rebellion, independence, heightened self-consciousness, experimentation, dating, driving, and concerns for the future. Conflicts over these issues often cause communication to break down between parents and children. You can work to avoid these conflicts by maintaining perspective and remaining sensitive to issues like peer pressure. He needs your support. Encourage open and honest discussion with your child regarding drugs, smoking, drinking, and sexually transmitted disease. Adolescents often know when they have done something wrong and can be embarrassed and frustrated by their actions. Let your child know that it's okay to talk with you.

Epilepsy can complicate this already fraught period. During adolescence, children face dramatic physical, mental, social, and academic changes. They feel a heightened sense of self-consciousness and exaggerated concerns over physical and social image, which can feed these fears. Even if your child's seizures are well controlled, these heightened emotions may cause him to be scared of social isolation or stigma related to disease. If his seizures have led to a restriction on his activities, this can accentuate the way he's different from his peers and cause added stress. Especially during these years, epilepsy can aggravate or create problems of low self-esteem, dependency, or behavioral difficulties. If your adolescent struggles with the personal and social impact of epilepsy, counseling can be very helpful.

Puberty

Puberty is the time when a person undergoes the sexual transition from childhood to adolescence. Sex hormones initiate these physical and mental changes. The age of puberty's onset varies considerably from person to person; children who go through puberty especially early or especially late are often concerned about the way this differentiates them from their peers, and they are sometimes teased about the differences in their bodies compared to their peers'.

As for how puberty affects a child with epilepsy, the sex hormones that come into play during this time affect a person's body and brain, altering electrical and chemical activity, personality, mood, and in some cases, seizure activity. In some children, seizures may begin or stop around puberty. The association can be coincidental. Scientific proof that the hormonal changes of puberty lead to the development or cessation of epilepsy is lacking. Once epilepsy develops, hormones such as estrogen can increase the likelihood of seizures, and many adolescent girls report that seizures often occur around their menstrual and ovulatory periods.

Rapid changes in growth and hormone levels during puberty can alter a child's antiepileptic drug (AED) blood levels. If your child's seizure control worsens around the time she's going through puberty, you'll want to consider the possibility that a decrease in AED levels is responsible.

Taking Medications

Rebellion and/or denial may dominate the psyche of adolescents, which is why it's not unusual for adolescents to resist and become less compliant about taking their medication. They can usually understand the consequences of not taking their AEDs, but often resist the medication in an effort to be "normal" and deny they have epilepsy. Along with your doctor, enlist your adolescent as an active partner in making treatment decisions and allow him to take greater responsibility for his own care. It may help if you allow your adolescent and doctor to be alone for part of each visit. This will foster independence, a sense of self-control, and trust between the doctor and the patient.

Ensure that your child is taking his medication. With older children and adolescents, the easiest and best assessment of compliance is simply to ask directly, "Are you taking your medication?" You can confirm whether your child is taking his medication regularly and reinforce his compliance by having his doctor measure his AED blood levels at intervals, and also by keeping an eye on your child's pill bottles at home. However, lower blood levels aren't a sure sign of noncompliance—as mentioned earlier, problems with drug absorption or metabolism, or a period of rapid growth in height and weight or elevated hormone levels, can cause lower AED levels.

Driving

Getting a driver's license is a milestone that most teenagers look forward to—a mark of independence. Although many people with epilepsy can drive, safety concerns and legal issues limit driving for others. In most states, a person with epilepsy must submit a letter or form from his doctor about his seizure disorder. Many states ask the doctor for a recommendation. The recommendation is influenced by the patient's compliance with his medication, so remind your adolescent that a favorable report depends on whether he takes his prescribed medications appropriately.

As the age for driving approaches, you'll need to review your child's medical history. If he's had no seizures for several years, with your doctor's consent you may want to lower and eventually stop medications. We recommend doing this at least six months before the driving age. If your child's seizures are poorly controlled as he approaches driving age, it may be time to ask for a referral to an epilepsy center for reevaluation and possible changes in therapy. Adolescents with uncontrolled seizures that affect consciousness or motor control cannot obtain a driver's license. For more specific information about driving and people with epilepsy, see Chapter 21.

Dating

Dating can be uncomfortable for all adolescents, and epilepsy can make a teen feel even more uneasy. One question your child may wonder about is when to tell someone he's dating about the disorder, and how to do so. Epilepsy should absolutely be discussed with anyone who your child is dating regularly, but it's fine—and actually reasonable—to wait until the relationship feels comfortable. If your adolescent's seizures are not well controlled, however, he'll need to discuss epilepsy with his dates sooner rather than later, and preferably in person.

This is another area in which an already emotional situation is often more challenging for a child with epilepsy. Everyone faces a fear of rejection when asking someone out on a date. A person with epilepsy, however, has the added fear of rejection *because* of having epilepsy. This fear is not completely unfounded. Some people hear the word *epilepsy* and become frightened, a reaction based on lack of knowledge. This is an additional reason that education is important. If your child is comfortable discussing epilepsy, the feelings and understanding of those around him (friends, dates, potential dates) will reflect that comfort. This doesn't mean your child won't be rejected. Rejection is part of dating. No one is immune. Although epilepsy is one of many possible reasons that one person may reject another, it is often not *the* reason.

Sexual Activity

As a relationship develops, intimate contact is the natural next step. There is no reason for your adolescent to fear having a seizure during kissing or other intimate contact any more than at other times. Intimate contact does not protect someone from a seizure, however. The more frequent your adolescent's seizures, the more likely a seizure will occur during intimate activity. Any partners should be educated about what to do if a seizure occurs.

Although the vast majority of people with epilepsy enjoy sexual feelings and activities, some find that they have less interest in sexual activity than their peers. Libido, or interest in sexual activity, may be affected by epilepsy or AEDs, especially those that activate liver enzymes. If this becomes an issue, it should be discussed with the patient's doctor, because changing medications or reducing the dosage can be helpful.

Use of Alcohol and Illegal Drugs

Adolescents are often exposed to alcohol and illegal drugs. Unfortunately, use of these substances often leads to trouble. Immaturity, impulsivity, and willingness to take chances place adolescents who use alcohol or other drugs in particularly dangerous situations, such as driving or sex. Alcohol is the leading cause of motor vehicle accidents in the United States, and teenage drivers in fatal accidents are more likely to have used alcohol than other age groups. Cocaine can cause strokes, heart attacks, seizures, or death.

The rules concerning alcohol use and epilepsy apply to both adolescents and adults, but greater caution as well as legal restrictions apply to the younger group. One or two alcoholic beverages usually cause no meaningful changes in AED levels or in seizure control. The problem is that one or two drinks tend to become three or four, and this leads to impaired judgment, more drinks, and more serious problems.

The main risk from excessive alcohol use is a withdrawal seizure. As alcohol levels start to decline in the brain, the depression of neuronal activity is lifted. But instead of a return to baseline, the brain cells "overshoot" and become hyperexcitable. This is the state in which a hangover occurs—and for people with epilepsy, this is a state that makes seizures more likely: the greater the depression (the more alcohol consumed), the greater the overshoot and tendency toward seizures.

Alcohol use also impairs restorative sleep and thus increases the tendency for seizures. Teenagers often sleep off their hangovers, and those with epilepsy may forget to take their bedtime and morning medications. Alcohol withdrawal, impaired sleep, and missed medication together create the perfect storm to produce seizures. Any one of these three factors can do it alone; together, the odds of a seizure increase greatly. Warn your adolescents that alcohol use can worsen seizure control. In addition, the combinations of AEDs and alcohol can be very sedating.

Cocaine has serious effects as well: It can cause seizures in someone who has never had them before and can worsen seizure control in someone with epilepsy. Seizures associated with cocaine use are much more dangerous than seizures that occur from other causes, and they can be fatal. Seizures can be caused or made worse by the use of stimulants, synthetic cannabis products, heroin or other opiates, LSD, PCP, ecstasy, or the withdrawal of sedative-anxiety drugs, such as benzodiazepines and barbiturates. Many of these drugs are illegal and all are potentially very dangerous for adolescents with epilepsy. As a whole, teenagers with epilepsy should not drink alcohol, smoke marijuana, or take other drugs. The role of compounds such as cannabidiol or tetrahydrocannabidiol or other cannabis (marijuana)-based therapies as AEDs remains uncertain. If some are effective, than intermittent use could potentially lead to withdrawal.

Thinking about a Career

Adolescents with well-controlled or infrequent seizures should have few or no limitations when it comes to choosing a career, but those with uncontrolled seizures may face some restrictions. Adolescents and adults with epilepsy—as well as those with developmental issues such as intellectual disability, cerebral palsy, or blindness—now have greater work opportunities. Yet it's critical to set realistic, while still progressive and positive, expectations with your child.

High school is a great time to start thinking about this future. Certain classes in high school or college can advance knowledge and skills related to your child's area of interest. Some children with epilepsy do not pursue college because of learning issues, and for them, high school is an especially critical time to prepare for adult life. Guidance counselors and vocational counselors often are available in high school to discuss career plans.

Part-Time Employment or Volunteering

Part-time work and volunteering can be rewarding for adolescents who have epilepsy. These opportunities can provide discipline, skills, education, and a sense of accomplishment and success. A part-time job or volunteer position is often a step toward independence. Help your adolescent choose an opportunity that's well balanced with his academic and social life and that won't cause sleep deprivation or work-related stress, since these issues can increase seizure frequency. Allow your child to take on responsibility. As your child grows through adolescence and into adulthood, present him with as many chances as possible to feel accomplished and independent.

18 | INTELLECTUAL AND BEHAVIORAL DEVELOPMENT

Most children with epilepsy are developmentally normal, with intellectual capacities typical for children their age and no behavioral issues. Many, however, do experience developmental delays that set them apart from others in their age group. These delays can be caused by genetic, metabolic, or structural brain disorders, as well antiepileptic drugs (AEDs), especially when the child is on multiple drugs or high doses. It's often difficult to determine the main cause of a child's developmental delays, because genetics, a physical or functional brain abnormality, seizures, or medications can all be involved. If your child's development is delayed, her physician should do an evaluation to determine the cause(s) to the extent possible, and should then develop a therapy plan that takes those delays into account. Some delays in children with epilepsy are reversible, and most are amenable to therapy, such as speech, physical, and occupational therapies.

The pace of any child's developmental progress is relative, so remember that almost all children develop to some degree, even if the pace is slower than the norm. Even children with severe cerebral palsy or severe intellectual disabilities grow and progress. We say "almost all," because in very rare cases of degenerative disorder, development can regress. For example, some children with epilepsy may lose previously attained milestones after a prolonged seizure, a cluster of seizures, or as a result of medication—but these children almost always recover and then continue to progress developmentally. There are cases in which a child may lose some speech and thinking abilities on one medication and then have that loss completely reversed after switching medications.

EFFECTS OF SEIZURES AND MEDICATION ON MENTAL FUNCTION

A single brief seizure will not cause permanent brain injury in a child with epilepsy, so when we talk about the long-term brain effects of seizures, we're referring to recurrent seizures. Even with recurrent seizures, which can have long-term effects, the effects vary from child to child and are not fully understood. Mild seizures—such as absence and simple partial seizures—do not injure the brain, but they may still affect the child's mental function. Children with these seizures may have higher rates of academic and social problems than typical children. This suggests that even in these mild and relatively benign epilepsies, cognition and behavior may sometimes be affected. Children with frequent complex partial seizures may have memory impairment and behavioral disorders. In these cases, it's not proven that the seizures themselves cause the problems. Many of these children also have structural abnormalities in areas of the brain that control memory or emotion, and these abnormalities are more likely at the root of the children's cognitive and behavioral difficulties.

The Effects of Frequent Tonic–Clonic Seizures

Children with frequent or prolonged tonic–clonic seizures often score lower on intelligence and memory tests than children without these seizures, suggesting that these particular seizures can be harmful. The negative mental effects are particularly apparent in people who've experienced a large number of the seizures or status epilepticus over many years. Again, these intellectual problems may be caused by the child's underlying brain disorder and not by the epilepsy. They may also be caused by recurrent seizures (especially tonic–clonic seizures), experiencing head injury, side effects of AEDs, and psychosocial factors. Any of these can play a role. Also, many children with epilepsy who were neurologically typical before the diagnosis of epilepsy have learning problems at the time that epilepsy is diagnosed; thus, the problems predate the epilepsy.

The Effect of AEDs on Intellect and Behavior

Our first pediatric neurologist told us that phenobarbital was like water, that we would never know that Brenda was on it. He was wrong. She became cranky, hyperactive, slept poorly—she was a different child. We were told this would pass, but it didn't. Our sweet child was gone, and another had taken her place. If we had to choose between the seizures and side effects, we would gladly take the seizures. The doctor we saw for a second opinion changed her medications. We had our daughter back. ■ ■ ■

Sally was just starting to speak—she had at least 12 words and was such a bright girl. Then she went on topiramate and it really affected her speech. Once we got her off it, she was back to normal. ■ ■ ■

Although the effect of frequent tonic–clonic seizures is often underestimated, parents often *overestimate* the negative effects of AEDs. Yes, AEDs can impair a child's intellectual performance and cause behavioral problems. However, among the primary AEDs used at standard doses (see Table 10.1), these effects are usually minor. In studies comparing intellectual functions while patients are on AEDs and then after they go off them, patients' cognitive functions overall improved only slightly or not at all after going off the drugs. As a result, it's safe to conclude that the drugs had little to no effect on the patients' intellect and behavioral issues. When AEDs do cause cognitive and behavioral changes it's often because the child is taking high doses. Children on high dosages of one or more AEDs are more likely to suffer side effects. There are exceptions: Some individuals may experience disabling problems as a result of a single AED, even at low doses.

As the dosage and blood levels of an AED increase, side effects also increase. With high blood levels, a child may experience excessive drowsiness and need for sleep, slowed thinking and movement, decreased initiative and motivation, memory lapses, and other cognitive deficits. Taking a combination of several AEDs also increases the likelihood that a child will have cognitive and other problems. When high doses or combinations of AED are used, it is worth considering the benefits of the drug or drugs versus the side effects. For example, you wouldn't want to increase the dosage of an AED—resulting in excessive tiredness and impaired academic performance—simply to reduce your child's complex partial seizures from three to two a month. The payoff is too small: The side effects would significantly impact your child's quality of life, whereas a complex partial seizure may disrupt only one to three minutes during the seizure and perhaps 20 minutes during its aftereffects.

Sometimes what you assume to be a negative effect of medication is actually something else: normal behavior for your child's age (temper tantrums in a two-year-old or irritability in a teenager, for example), social issues, seizures, underlying brain disorders, or other factors. Your parental observations, as well as reports from teachers and others who are close to your child, can help determine the cause of any problems. Be sure to carefully document any side effects and their relationship to when the medication was taken. And be aware that when a child has taken AEDs for years, it is often difficult to distinguish medication effects from "who the child is." Even older children, if they've been on medication for a long time, may not be able to remember what it was like to be off medications. Lowering, discontinuing, or switching medications may be the only way to find out if behavioral changes result from the drugs or are a feature of your child's personality.

As discussed in Chapter 9, "Principles of Drug Therapy for Epilepsy," side effects and seizures can often be reduced by changing the timing of your child's doses. An immediate-release medication can be given after meals to minimize peak side effects caused by rapid absorption of the drug, for example. When available, extended-release forms of the medication maintain steadier levels, reducing side effects and improving seizure control. In other cases, more frequent but smaller doses can help to maintain steadier blood levels of the drug.

BEHAVIORAL AND LEARNING PROBLEMS

Behavioral problems can occur around the time your child experiences seizures. This section looks at problems that are not unique to children with epilepsy but that occur at increased rates in the epilepsy population. We'll discuss learning disorders, difficulty with concentration (attention deficit), hyperactivity, and language and cognitive impairments, as well as anxiety, irritability, aggressive verbal or physical behavior, depression, mood swings, poor social skills, lack of motivation and energy, and inability to plan or organize behavior.

Learning Disorders

In children with learning disorders, there is a discrepancy between the child's intellectual level and academic achievement; that is, the child's intelligence outpaces her achievement. Neurological disorders such as epilepsy can cause learning disorders, but most children with epilepsy do not have learning disorders.

Learning requires a complicated series of brain processes. To absorb information, your child must pay attention and perceive (see and/or hear the material). If she cannot pay attention or perceive properly, she cannot learn effectively. Memory involves her actively comparing newly acquired information with previously learned information, and then recalling it when necessary. These are only a few of the many complex steps in the process of learning.

The most extensively studied learning disorder is dyslexia, a developmental reading disorder. Dyslexia's cause is not understood, but the brain's left temporal and parietal lobes—areas critical for reading and language comprehension—are involved. Seizures can affect these areas. Still, this doesn't mean that in a child with both epilepsy and dyslexia, the two disorders are related. Reading can be impaired by many kinds of problems. Children who cannot focus their attention for more than a few seconds may have secondary reading problems. Visual problems can impair reading. Reading can also be disrupted by right (nonlanguage-dominant) hemisphere brain disorders that interfere with a child's ability to scan and see the left side of a page or the left side of words.

Other learning problems affect arithmetic, spoken information, visual information other than reading, relating visual information to movement components (visuomotor disorders), and relating objects in space (disorders of visuospatial analysis). Some children have difficulty understanding social rules and emotionally relating to peers or adults. These problems are more common among children with epilepsy, and depend on many factors, including the location of the seizure focus, seizure frequency, and medication side effects. However, in some cases these learning problems may be coincidental and not related to epilepsy.

If you suspect that your child has a learning disability, you should request that she be evaluated by a school psychologist, neuropsychologist, or child study team. Such services can be requested through your child's school. The evaluation can often identify the type of and cause of a learning disorder.

Severe Language, Cognitive, and Behavioral Impairments

Some children with epilepsy have severe language and cognitive impairments. This can be a result of other social and behavioral problems that are present in these children, since socializing is the primary way that children obtain language skills. Similarly, language impairment can severely hinder a child's social interactions—so it becomes an escalating spiral. In this section we discuss some of the impairments most common in children with epilepsy.

Attention Deficit Disorder

Attention is the foundation on which intellectual functions rest. If you do not pay attention, you cannot efficiently understand, learn, or remember information. Attention involves a filtering process preventing the mind from becoming overwhelmed by too many images, sensations, and feelings and thoughts. The attentional filtering system develops in children around the time that fine movement control and ability to learn abstract mathematical relationships also develop. A three-year-old simply cannot sit quietly for a few hours and work on a puzzle.

Attention deficit disorder (ADD) is a common problem in schoolchildren, characterized by poor concentration, distractibility, impulsivity, and an inability to maintain attention. These may seem like problems you'd see in all young children, but in children with ADD, the levels of these issues exceed the norm. Because these issues interfere with learning, teachers as well as parents frequently notice them. ADD usually begins before the age of five and is more common in boys. Hyperactivity (discussed in the "Hyperactivity" subsection) and ADD often coexist in the same child, and this is referred to as *attention deficit hyperactivity disorder (ADHD)*. The two disorders are separate, however, and one may occur without the other. ADD refers to cognitive behavior, whereas hyperactivity refers to motor behavior. Children with epilepsy have higher incidences of both ADD and hyperactivity. In some children with epilepsy, the attention and hyperactivity problems are related to the underlying neurological problem that causes their seizures.

The root cause of ADD/ADHD is unknown. Parents of some children report that consumption of sugar noticeably reduces their children's attention spans. Some of these parents choose to limit their children's sugar consumption. Medical studies, however, have generally not found dietary restrictions to improve ADD/ADHD symptoms. The only restriction that has shown some effect is eliminating foods with colorings and additives for children with food sensitivities. As far as we know, ADD may be a disorder of brain maturity or a chemical imbalance. In most children, the impact of ADD lessens as they mature, with fewer problems arising in adolescence, although 40 percent of cases persist into adulthood.

Medications can cause or accentuate attention deficit, since any drug that makes a person tired can impair attention. In addition, barbiturates, benzodiazepines, and levetiracetam can cause hyperactivity, which also impairs attention. Topiramate can impair attention and mental processing speed. Because all seizure medications alter the brain's electrical or chemical function, there is a potential that these drugs may affect your child's attention or other cognitive functions. In many cases, by reducing seizures and epilepsy waves between seizures, these medications actually improve attention. If attention problems develop or worsen after a drug is started or the dosage is increased, however, be sure to inform your doctor. In some cases, the problem may lessen within weeks or a few months; in other cases, the dosage may have to be reduced or the medication changed.

Treating Attention Deficit Disorder in Children with Epilepsy

When ADD causes learning or social problems, medical therapy can be helpful. Behavioral modification is of limited benefit for children with ADD and has proven less effective than medication. The drugs used to treat ADD include stimulants, atomoxetine (Strattera), and guanfacine (Tenex and the extended release Intuniv). In children with ADD, stimulants paradoxically lead to a more relaxed and focused state of mind. The most commonly used stimulants are methylphenidate (Ritalin, Concerta, Metadate, Methylin, Daytrana), demethylphenidate (Focalin), and amphetamines (Adderall and Vyvanse). These drugs can be used safely in children for prolonged periods, but must be carefully supervised by a doctor. Side effects include decreased appetite and weight loss, stomach discomfort, difficulty sleeping, depression, and irritability. Long-term use may lead to a slight decrease in growth. Many children require lower doses as they grow older and can eventually come off ADD mediations.

In the vast majority of children with epilepsy over age three years, stimulant drugs can be used safely. Keep in mind that insomnia, a potential side effect of stimulants, can increase seizure activity. Although a particular stimulant, methylphenidate, is listed in the *Physician's Drug Reference* as a rare cause of worsening seizures, there is very little evidence to support this claim. The majority of children with epilepsy and ADD/ADHD, however, experience improved attention with no worsening of seizure control after going on a stimulant. Many children are able to skip their stimulants on weekends and vacations.

Atomoxetine and guanfacine are nonstimulant alternatives to treat ADD/ADHD. They can be safely used in epilepsy patients and have fewer side effects (no appetite or growth suppression, less insomnia than stimulants), but many people find them less effective than stimulants. Working with your child's doctor, you may find it helpful to combine one of these medications with a stimulant.

Impulsivity is a feature of ADD that can affect a child's social relations and academic achievements. *Impulsivity* refers to a person's tendency to act automatically in response to environmental stimuli, without considering the consequences of those actions. Stimulants, atomoxetine, and clonidine (Catapres) can reduce impulsivity. Clonidine can cause sedation but does not worsen seizure control in children with epilepsy.

Hyperactivity

Children as a whole are much more physically active than adults. In some children, excessive movement, or hyperactivity, causes problems. The increased activity can take several forms: excessive fidgeting, an inability to stay seated for more than a minute, and/or running around endlessly. Hyperactivity causes problems because it prevents the child from staying in one place and can disrupt the classroom and home. Hyperactivity is most often seen in boys.

Hyperactivity is significantly more common among children with epilepsy. It is also more common among children with tic disorders. The drugs that can improve ADD can also treat hyperactivity.

OTHER PSYCHIATRIC DISORDERS

Children with epilepsy suffer higher rates of depression, anxiety, and irritability, as well as more serious mental disorders. These psychological problems may be unrelated to epilepsy or may be influenced by the child's emotional reactions to having epilepsy, the effect of medications, the underlying cause of the child's epilepsy (such as head trauma), or the epilepsy itself.

The behavioral changes associated with psychological disorders can occur around the time of a seizure (peri-ictal, which means happening before, during, or after a seizure) or during the interval between seizures (interictal). Some individuals and family members report symptoms such as irritability or sadness occurring hours or even days before a seizure. It's common for children to feel emotions—most often fear and anxiety—during partial seizures, for example. After a complex partial or tonic–clonic seizure, children may experience depression, irritability, anxiety, or hyperactivity. If the complex partial or tonic–clonic seizures are prolonged or occur in a cluster, behavioral changes can be more pronounced and rarely include psychosis. (*Psychosis* refers to a serious disorder of thought in which the patient's "connection to reality" is impaired; paranoia, delusions, or hallucinations may be involved.)

Most of the behavioral changes discussed in this section occur interictally—between seizures. The changes occur as relatively stable patterns of behavior.

Personality Changes

Some children with epilepsy undergo personality changes in which the pattern of their thinking, feeling, and behaving is altered. Because everyone's personality evolves over childhood and adolescence, it is very difficult to study the effects of epilepsy on this dynamic characteristic.

There's currently some debate about whether certain traits are more frequent in people with temporal lobe epilepsy than those with other forms of focal epilepsy or generalized epilepsy. Because the temporal and frontal lobes both contain areas that control emotional and social functions, as well as other areas that determine executive skills (judgment, reasoning) and personality (especially frontal lobe), any disorder (head trauma, epilepsy, stroke, etc.) affecting these areas could potentially alter behavior.

Generalized epilepsies, such as juvenile myoclonic epilepsy, are also associated with an increased frequency of psychiatric disorders, such as depression, anxiety, impairments in executive functions, and personality changes. However, many children with generalized epilepsies do not have behavioral problems. And although generalized epilepsies are fundamentally different from partial epilepsies, they also involve the brain's frontal and temporal regions, as well as other cortical and subcortical regions. Coexisting disorders contribute to a high rate of long-term adult psychosocial problems. Once, absence epilepsy was considered cognitively and behaviorally benign. Then a well-designed study compared children with absence epilepsy to those with juvenile rheumatoid arthritis (to control for the effects of chronic illness) at a follow-up after age 18. The children with absence epilepsy had greater difficulties with academic, personal, and behavioral functioning.

When personality or behavioral changes interfere with your child's personal, family, or school life, seek help. Your doctor's office can work with you to find the right professionals to help you deal with these issues.

Irritability

Children with epilepsy may be more prone toward irritability. There are a number of reasons for this. Irritability is commonly caused by stress and tiredness, but may also be influenced by medications such as phenobarbital, levetiracetam, zonisamide, and benzodiazepines, as well as brain abnormalities in areas that regulate emotions, and possibly by the epilepsy itself. You may notice that irritability precedes or follows your child's seizures.

A change in medications or improved seizure control may reduce your child's anxiety and irritability. If your child is one of the few with epilepsy in whom irritability is a serious problem, discuss it with the doctor. A change in AED or dosage, treatment of an underlying depression or sleep disorder, or psychotherapy may prove beneficial. Buspirone and selective serotonin re uptake inhibitors can also help when warranted. In more serious cases, low doses of antipsychotic medications may be used.

Aggression

The vast majority of children with epilepsy are no more aggressive than those in the general population, but some do show excessive aggressive behavior. This may be related to AEDs, underlying brain abnormalities, epilepsy, or the confused state some patients experience after seizures. Children naturally have less impulse control than adults, and they reflexively translate thoughts into actions. Control over social behavior and aggressive impulses is acquired progressively during childhood.

Certain medications can make aggressive behavior more likely to occur, especially in predisposed individuals. Barbiturates, benzodiazepines, and levetiracetam are most likely to cause aggressive behaviors.

During a seizure, directed aggressive behavior is exceedingly rare, but aggressive behavior can occur during the period of confusion after a tonic–clonic seizure, usually because someone tries to restrain the person. The best response to such a reaction is to remove the restraint.

Depression

Depression is a major factor impairing the quality of life of children with epilepsy. Depression causes feelings of sadness, helplessness, hopelessness, and guilt, and it impairs a child's ability to experience happiness. The borderline between sadness and depression is imprecise, but when sadness is prolonged and causes a sustained impairment in a child's ability to enjoy life and school, there is a problem. Many depressed children also suffer from insomnia or sleep excessively.

The most serious complication of depression is suicide, and adolescents with epilepsy, especially those older than age 15, show a slightly increased rate of suicide. Patients, family members, and doctors often fail to recognize the presence or severity of depression. If you have any suspicion that your child may suffer from depression, seek help. Any child or adolescent who expresses thoughts about hurting himself should be taken extremely seriously, and a psychiatrist or other appropriate mental health worker should be consulted.

Causes of Depression

Depression can stem from a child's psychological reaction to having epilepsy; from medication effects; from the cause of the epilepsy or from the epilepsy itself. The relative importance of each of these factors varies from case to case, and often several factors coexist. If the psychological effects of living with epilepsy caused the depression, it often improves when the person discusses her troublesome feelings with a therapist. Antiepileptic medications and other drugs (such as steroids) can cause depression—and in these cases, it is often dose-related; that is, the higher the dose, the greater the risk and severity of depression.

Treatment of Depression

When possible, the cause or causes should be addressed. Serious depression requires treatment that can include therapy (such as cognitive behavioral or psychotherapy) and antidepressant medication. Some doctors fear that antidepressants (such as selective serotonin and serotonin/norepinephrine reuptake inhibitors) can aggravate a seizure disorder. However, antidepressant medications are more likely to improve seizure control, possibly by improving mood and restorative sleep, and reducing stress.

Anxiety

All people experience anxiety and nervousness to some degree. It becomes a disorder when the anxious feelings are frequent or intense, are produced by trivial things or by nothing at all, and interfere with functioning. Anxiety disorders are more common among children with epilepsy than children without epilepsy. Several factors can cause anxiety disorders in children with epilepsy, including psychological stress related to having epilepsy or other issues, medication effects, associated neurological or psychiatric disorders, and the epilepsy itself. However, in many cases, the anxiety predates the epilepsy, and they may share some common underlying mechanisms.

Anxiety disorders can be effectively treated with counseling, therapy, and medications. Buspirone, selective serotonin and serotonin/norepinephrine reuptake inhibitors are safe for almost all patients with epilepsy and anxiety.

Benzodiazepines are very effective in the short-term treatment of anxiety and insomnia, but they should be avoided for long-term use. Over time, they often lose effectiveness and may contribute to cognitive and behavioral problems. Benzodiazepines commonly used to treat anxiety include clonazepam (Klonopin), diazepam (Valium), alprazolam (Xanax), and lorazepam (Ativan). These drugs can also temporarily reduce seizure frequency and intensity, but after a period of weeks, the effect on anxiety, insomnia, and seizure control diminishes. As the original anxiety or seizures return, there's a strong tendency for patients and doctors to increase the dose, which again briefly reduces troublesome symptoms. This cycle leads to a dangerous buildup of the dose, leading to levels that can cause memory impairment, depression, tiredness, and other problems. If the dose is then reduced, the real trouble begins: anxiety, insomnia, and seizures become more severe. Clobazam (Onfi) is an exception to this cycle and can provide long-term improvement in seizure control for many children, but has not been shown to have sustained effectiveness in treating anxiety.

Autism Spectrum Disorders (ASD or Autism)

Autism is a persistent disorder that begins in the first three years of a child's life and that affects social communication and interaction. Children with autism display restricted, repetitive patterns of behavior and interests. They often make little eye contact, do not interact normally with people in their environment, and show a wide spectrum of cognitive and behavioral problems. Among all children with autism, approximately 25 percent will develop epilepsy by the time they turn 20 years old. Among children whose seizures begin in the first two years of life, autism develops in up to 15 percent. For babies with infantile spasms, more than 30 percent will develop autism.

The overlaps between epilepsy and autism are complex and include genetic and environmental factors. We now know of multiple genes (for example, those that cause tuberous sclerosis, Dravet syndrome, duplication 15q syndrome, and Fragile X) that cause both epilepsy and autism. In children with epilepsy and autism, the goal is to treat both disorders.

Psychosis

Psychosis is a serious mental disorder in which a person suffers from impaired content and coherence of thoughts, reduced connection to reality, and paranoia. A child or adolescent suffering from psychosis may experience delusions or disturbances of perception (hallucinations and distortions of sensation), or extremes of emotions. If a child who has recently shown her first symptoms of epilepsy develops psychosis or other prominent behavioral changes, the child's physician should consider whether the child has an autoimmune epilepsy syndrome such as anti-VGKC, anti-GABAB, anti-VGCC, and anti-GAD65 (see Chapter 4).

Psychosis can occur between seizures or after a cluster of complex partial or tonic–clonic seizures. People whose psychosis comes on after seizures often appear well for a few hours or days after the seizures, and then express disordered thoughts, delusional ideas, and aggressive behavior. Such psychoses can be effectively treated with antipsychotic drugs and benzodiazepines. Prompt recognition and treatment are critical.

Newer antipsychotic drugs rarely worsen seizure control. These drugs include quetiapine (Seroquel), risperidone (Risperdal), olanzapine (Zyprexa), aripiprazole (Abilify), and ziprasidone (Geodon).

UNUSUAL SEIZURES WITH PSYCHOLOGICAL SYMPTOMS

Some children with epilepsy, especially those with focal seizures, may experience unusual and bizarre phenomena during seizures that affect their intellectual or behavioral functioning. The experiences can be fascinating, frightening, or both. Very often, children are reluctant to discuss strange symptoms or experiences because they cannot put them into words, fear being considered crazy, or because they are used to these symptoms and consider them a part of who they are. However, symptoms that begin suddenly and last for a brief time can be seizures no matter how strange they seem.

The following are descriptions patients have given of unusual seizures, often provided only after specific questions were asked:

- "I had a feeling of extreme embarrassment, as though I had made a very foolish remark."
- "I feel that someone else is in the room behind me, that I am not alone."
- "Looking into the mirror, I noticed that the right side of my face was missing."
- "On the left half of space I saw colored balls of light. As I looked at them, they changed to multiple figures of small men. On later occasions, I recognized these as myself—tiny replicas that would approach and then recede."
- "I have a flood of thoughts; I don't know where they come from; I can't shut them off."
- " My seizures start with fear, and then I feel as if I am a character in the video game and the monster is going to eat me. I feel like I am in the machine."
- "The next thing I knew I was floating just below the ceiling."

While these experiences are not typical symptoms of seizures, the range of seizure symptoms is extremely broad; almost any emotion or experience is possible. As with most seizure symptoms, the emotional experiences described in the preceding list are brief, lasting less than three minutes, though on rare occasions they can last longer. The feature that helps classify them as epileptic and not a purely psychological issue is their sudden onset, although symptoms and experiences unrelated to epilepsy can be brief and begin suddenly.

Children and adolescents who experience phenomena such as the ones described should mention them to their parents and doctor. If the symptoms precede definite complex partial or tonic–clonic seizures, then they are very likely part of the seizure (a simple partial seizure).

We've discussed a wide range of behavioral and intellectual issues related to epilepsy in this chapter. But many children with epilepsy don't encounter any of these issues. And many of the issues are easily treatable or will be grown out of with time.

19 | EDUCATION AND CHILDREN WITH EPILEPSY

Most children with epilepsy have normal intelligence and keep up with their peers in school, but some do not. If your child is doing well in school, there is no reason to worry about the effects of epilepsy on his learning. If you notice that your child is lagging academically, however, it's important to find out why. An underlying neurological disorder—a genetic abnormality or prior head trauma, frequent seizures, or side effects of AEDs—can affect school performance. If your child's teacher reports problems or if you notice an academic problem yourself, the first step is to identify the problem. Your child may be experiencing attention deficit and distractibility; the problem may be excessive tiredness from medications or poor sleep; or it may be the result of a specific learning disability. The learning disability may or may not be related to the epilepsy (see Chapter 18). The best way to make this determination is through an educational assessment. Parents have the right to request an assessment of their child's problems and needs, and if you think one is warranted, talk to your child's teachers.

The Individuals with Disabilities Education Act (IDEA), discussed later, provides legal guarantees pertaining to the education of children with handicaps. Like all children, your child has the right to be taught in a regular classroom environment to the extent possible—Free and Appropriate Public Education (FAPE; Section 504 of the Rehabilitation Act of 1973). Your child has the right to be included in social and other activities provided by the school. Parents have the right to be directly involved in planning their child's education.

ATTENDING REGULAR CLASSES

Most children with epilepsy attend regular classes, even if in some cases they need special aides to work them. Regular classes offer an opportunity for children with epilepsy and other disorders to enjoy their education and to be in a social environment with their peers. Mainstream classes expose children to a wider array of social and academic opportunities and foster the feeling of being a kid, rather than of being a child with a disability. Some children in these regular classes may not be able to fully keep up, but they can gain tremendously in the emotional, social, and academic areas if you emphasize not just their achievements, but also their potential to learn and to accomplish the things that other children can.

Social and academic problems may arise for children with epilepsy who attend regular classes, so keep an eye on how your child is doing. Children can be cruel; teasing, excluding other children, bullying and cyberbullying are not unusual. Rarely, other parents may even forbid their children to play with a child who has epilepsy. If problems occur at school, consider asking the school to conduct an educational program so that your child's classmates can better understand epilepsy. Often these exclusionary feelings stem from a lack of knowledge about epilepsy.

SPECIAL EDUCATION

Special education programs are school-based programs designed to meet the needs of children with disabilities by supplementing or adapting the regular curriculum. Instruction in these programs may take place in regular classrooms or in separate facilities for all or part of the day. Students may also be assigned to special programs in physical education, occupational and physical rehabilitation, music education, home instruction, or instruction in hospitals and other institutions.

If your child is not doing well in his mainstream classes, you should meet with his teachers to identify the problems. A comprehensive evaluation (medical, neurological, educational, neuropsychological), and communication between the various parties (teachers, parents, doctors, testing professionals) may help identify the cause. In some cases the critical information can come from vision or hearing tests, or psychiatric or other assessments.

Schools are required to deliver services for your child in the "least restrictive environment," meaning the regular classroom for as much of the day as possible. Some children require many special classes or even a special school, and emotional issues can arise when children are removed from the mainstream. If your child is educated in a special class or school, you'll want to be aware that other special needs children in the class may have emotional or behavioral problems and can thus provide poor behavioral models. If this becomes a problem, talk with teachers or school administrators. You and your child's teachers should always emphasize that your child is special, not handicapped, disabled, or less bright. You and the teachers should not deny or avoid discussing your child's epilepsy or other disabilities, but should emphasize the positive.

INDIVIDUALS WITH DISABILITIES ACT

The IDEA ensures that all disabled children receive appropriate education at no cost and, as mentioned earlier, in the least restrictive environment. All states that receive federal funds under this act must follow the rules for identifying, evaluating, and providing services to eligible children between 3 and 21 years of age. Federal funds are also provided to the states to develop early intervention services for infants and toddlers with physical or mental conditions that are likely to cause developmental delay.

This act recognizes the special needs of children with disabilities, including children with epilepsy, intellectual disabilities, hearing and visual impairments (not limited to deafness and blindness), autism, serious emotional disorders, orthopedic impairments, traumatic brain injury, learning disabilities, and other impairments that require special education and related services. A child who only has epilepsy may qualify if the disorder affects the child's educational capacity to the degree that special education or related services are required.

Some children with epilepsy may have problems that require special attention even if their seizures are not disabling and their intelligence is normal. These include impairments of attention, reading, arithmetic learning, motor skills, memory, and behavior. These impairments are often identified at a young age, permitting early intervention and treatment.

IDEA's "least restrictive environment" requirement specifically means that your child has the right to be educated in a classroom with children who do not have disabilities, to the maximum extent that this placement meets your child's educational needs. IDEA also requires that schools provide all the additional services needed to help children with disabilities benefit from special education. These services include transportation, audiology and speech therapy, psychological evaluation and treatment, physical and occupational therapy, recreation, therapeutic recreation, social work services, counseling, early identification and assessment of disabling conditions, and medical evaluations.

For children with epilepsy, related services include education for teachers and school nurses about epilepsy, plus training in how to administer medications and first aid for seizures. Ideally, this education will be extended to include your child's classmates, because social acceptance remains a challenge.

IDEA states that a child with disabilities must have a written individualized educational plan (IEP) constructed jointly by the parents and school personnel. The IEP is a written report describing your child's present level of development, short-term and annual goals of the special education program, specific educational services your child will receive, the date services will start for your child and their expected duration, standards for determining whether the goals of the educational program are being met, and the extent to which your child can participate in regular educational programs.

THE REHABILITATION ACT OF 1973, SECTION 504

Section 504 of the Rehabilitation Act of 1973 provides education rights for children and adults with disabilities. This antidiscrimination law makes it illegal for any program or activity receiving federal funding to exclude or discriminate against qualified people with handicaps. It also requires that educational institutions make reasonable accommodations.

Section 504 covers "qualified" people with handicaps—not only children of school age, but also adult educational services that may include college, graduate school, and technical schools.

20 | CAMPS AND SPORTS

Alli has played soccer since she was five years old. Can she still play now that she has had a seizure? What about summer camp? I want her life to be as full as possible. ■ ■ ■

As important as school is, it's not the only arena where your child has the opportunity to build relationships with other children of the same age. Sports are a vital part of childhood and offer crucial opportunities for kids to learn teamwork, sharing, self-discipline, and skills that can help in the development of personality, confidence, and character. Children's athletic abilities and interest in sports vary greatly, but there's no reason for a child with epilepsy who is interested in athletics to be deprived of the opportunity. If your child is interested, she should be encouraged to participate in group and competitive sports, such as community teams, Little League baseball, and school sports. These activities are usually well supervised and require appropriate safety gear. For those children who do enjoy group activities, individual sports, or exercise programs, we encourage participation as it promotes a healthy body weight. Serious injuries in children with epilepsy are uncommon and infrequently occur during participation in sports.

Summer camps, as well as organizations such as Scouts, clubs, and religious groups, can foster social development. For children with epilepsy, the decision to participate in an activity should be individualized and should involve discussions between the child and parent. A child's types of seizures and frequency are critical in determining which sports and activities are safe. Children who have uncontrolled, frequent seizures should know that certain activities are restricted. For example, they should not swim alone (in fact, *no* child should swim alone), or play on high bars or climb ropes without a proper mat and supervision.

CAMP LIFE

All children with epilepsy can enjoy camp. If your child's seizures are well controlled or infrequent, she should have no problem attending any regular camp. You'll need to speak with the camp management and counselors about the range of activities appropriate for your child and any precautions that must be taken. Most children with epilepsy enjoy very full and active camp experiences with little restriction. Children who have more frequent seizures or who have not met other children with seizures may benefit from going to a camp where there are other children who have epilepsy. Epilepsy.com and your local epilepsy foundation can provide information about these camps. Scholarships may be available from organizations such as Finding a Cure for Epilepsy and Seizures (FACES). Some camps specialize in programs for children with severe epilepsy, cerebral palsy, or emotional disorders. These camps provide a wonderful social opportunity for children and an invaluable respite for their parents.

WATER SPORTS AND SWIMMING

Water—lakes, oceans, ponds, rivers, streams, pools—can be dangerous for any child. No child, regardless of whether they have seizures, should swim alone. A child who has ongoing seizures that impair motor control or consciousness should only swim when under close supervision. Swimming pools are considerably safer than open water such as lakes or the ocean, where a child can easily escape the sight of a supervisor and can be difficult to locate quickly in an emergency situation. Even in a pool setting, your child should consider swimming with a "buddy," and you'll want to make sure a responsible lifeguard is on duty who knows that a child at risk for seizures is in the water. When swimming in a lake, bay, or ocean life jackets are recommended to ensure safety, since the tide can make it difficult to reach a child quickly in the event that she has a seizure while swimming. Note that children with absence seizures also sink during a seizure.

When a child with epilepsy is in a boat, the main risk is that she will fall into the water. A child who is sailing may be knocked into the water by the boom. All children in boats should wear life jackets.

Older children whose seizures are well controlled can snorkel and may even scuba dive. Children with uncontrolled seizures that impair consciousness or motor control should not scuba dive and should only snorkel in relatively calm water, close to someone who has life saving skills.

You know your child best and will need to keep your child's particular needs in mind when selecting water sports and activities. The most important factors whenever you're around water are supervision and proper precautions. As long as you or another responsible party is watching your child closely, your child can enjoy the water with minimal risk of harm.

BICYCLING

Bicycling near the street or a high traffic area can pose a serious danger for people with uncontrolled seizures. Even if a parent rides close by the child, a seizure can suddenly cause the child to veer into traffic and fall. If your child has uncontrolled seizures, be sure to ride only in nontraffic zones such as a park or designated bike trail. Children with controlled seizures or whose seizures do not impair motor control or consciousness can ride bikes unrestricted.

Stationary exercise bikes pose no serious danger for children with epilepsy. Ideally, the floor beneath the bike should be carpeted or padded in case your child falls off. Low-seated bicycles are safest.

HORSEBACK RIDING

Horseback riding can be safe and fun for children whose seizures are well controlled or are usually preceded by a warning sign. Even children who have seizures that can cause them to fall off a horse can ride with supervision. While the child is riding, an adult should walk close beside the horse to make sure the rider is safe in the event of a fall. Competitive horseback riding, which involves galloping and jumping, should be considered only if your child's epilepsy is well controlled.

CONTACT SPORTS

Football, basketball, soccer, rugby, ice hockey, and lacrosse are generally safe for people with epilepsy. The principal concern for all children taking part in contact sports is the risk of head or bodily injury. However children with epilepsy are at little or no increased risk of injury than any other child. Tackle football, rugby, and ice hockey have a higher incidence of injuries than most other sports and participation in these should be limited to children with well-controlled seizures. This doesn't mean children with epilepsy can't play some form of these games. For example, a child who has occasional or even frequent seizures can play touch football or a lower-contact version of these other activities. Helmets should be worn when playing sports such as football, ice hockey, and baseball batting. Wrestling may be safe for children with well-controlled seizures, or seizures that do not impair motor control and consciousness. Similarly, gymnastics can be safe for children with epilepsy, but this depends on the specific gymnastic activity. The high bar, uneven parallel bars, balance beam, and vault can be dangerous for children with ongoing seizures, given the risk of falling, but can be safe for those with well-controlled seizures. Other gymnastic events such as the pommel horse and floor routine pose less risk and can usually be enjoyed by all with spotting when needed.

TELLING THE COACH

Both you and your child should be honest with coaches involved in your child's sports. This is the only way adequate supervision and preparation can be made to ensure your child's safety. A seizure action plan should be discussed and implemented so that the coach will be prepared if a seizure occurs. For rescue medication, a parent or caretaker can be in the stands and administer the treatment as needed. When the proper precautions are taken and the proper notifications and plans made, there's no reason most children with epilepsy can't enjoy the same kinds of active fun as their peers. As your child moves from childhood into adolescence and then adulthood, she can continue to participate in sports and continue to feel a part of the greater community.

21 YOUR CHILD'S FUTURE WITH EPILEPSY: DRIVING, WORK, MARRIAGE, PARENTHOOD

As children with epilepsy transition out of adolescence and into adulthood, they'll be faced with decisions about driving, employment, and other activities. If their seizures are rare or fully controlled, they'll be able to safely pursue most activities. If they have frequent seizures that impair consciousness, some activities such as driving will not be possible until seizures can hopefully be controlled for a sustained period.

RISK-BENEFIT DECISIONS

High-risk activities like skydiving, scuba diving, motorcycle riding, or fighting fires can potentially cause injury or death, yet millions of people voluntarily participate in them every year. They do so because they feel that the benefits—enjoyment, employment, or helping others—outweigh the risks. Many more of us engage in lower-risk activities that can pose a danger, such as driving a car, biking on roads, or snorkeling.

In weighing the risks versus benefits for people with epilepsy, the decisions are heavily influenced by the person's level of seizure control. If the person's seizures are well controlled, the risk-benefit equation of a particular activity will mirror that same equation for a person without epilepsy. For people with frequent, uncontrolled seizures, activities such as swimming and bike riding can be carried out with precautions, but other activities such as driving are unsafe and can endanger other people as well as the person with epilepsy. The most difficult decisions involve persons who have occasional seizures. In these cases, it's important to weigh all the risks for the person with the seizures, as well as risk to other people, and also the benefit to that person's quality of life that the activity in question would bring.

QUALITY OF LIFE

The concept of "quality of life" is relatively new in medicine and involves the patient's, not the doctor's, perspective on an illness and how it affects daily living. Although it would seem that a patient's and doctor's views would be similar in this area, they can be quite different. Quality-of-life studies are giving us new insights into the effect of disorders and treatments and into ways of improving patients' lives.

For example, some doctors consider occasional seizures acceptable and minor medication side effects tolerable. (Of course, in some cases, seizures cannot be fully controlled, and side effects invariably occur despite the doctor's best attempts to adjust the medications.) These doctors might not aggressively try to control the seizures further or might not attempt to reduce the side effects— based on their own perceptions of what is acceptable to the patient. But what they're not taking into account are the patient's perceptions. Often the doctor does not see a problem worthy of attention, but the patient does. This is a gap in communication. The person who has occasional seizures may appear fine, but could be facing restrictions or problems with driving, employment, finances, social and family life, and self-esteem. Fear of another seizure may be the person's greatest disability. To the patient, these seizures that appear tolerable to the doctor are creating real-life havoc.

Achieving the best quality of life is a challenge. Tolerating an occasional seizure may be better than daily side effects needed for full control; other patients prefer the cost of full control, especially if that full control allows them to take part in more activities. There is no right answer here; dialogue between patient and doctor is the key to finding the right balance. In this dialogue, the doctor needs to work hard to pay attention to the patient's expectations and actual experience of living with epilepsy. In turn, the patient must help her doctors understand how epilepsy and its treatment are affecting her life.

MOTOR-VEHICLE DRIVING

For many people, a driver's license is a passport to adulthood. In addition to the emotional satisfaction of passing the driving test, in rural and suburban areas driving can be essential for independence and employment. Driving is a privilege, however, and applicants for a license must meet all of their state's criteria to qualify for a driver's license. Applicants in all states must be older than a minimum age; must pass a written test, a vision test, and a driving test; and must not have a medical disorder that would make driving dangerous.

Licensure of People with Epilepsy

State laws determine which medical conditions disqualify someone from obtaining a driver's license. These laws protect public safety and grant the privilege of driving to people who are the least likely to have an accident.

What does this mean for people with epilepsy? Seizures that impair consciousness or motor control can cause serious accidents. As a result, the rate of motor vehicle accidents for people with epilepsy is higher than average, but it's much lower than the accident rate for people who've been drinking alcohol above the legal limit. In some cases, accidents involving epilepsy are caused by people, especially men, who drive without a license or who fail to report their epilepsy when applying for a license.

To obtain a driver's license in most states, a person with epilepsy must be free of seizures that affect consciousness and motor control, must have been free of these seizures for a certain period, and must submit a doctor's statement of opinion that the person can drive safely. The seizure-free period usually varies from three months to one year, but many states consider exceptions that will permit someone to drive after a shorter interval.

The Review and Decision Process

A state's department of motor vehicles reviews medical information and in complex cases often forwards the information to a consulting doctor or medical advisory board. Most states have such a board, which may also hear appeals concerning decisions to deny or revoke drivers' licenses.

Some states allow people who have persistent seizures to drive if those seizures do not impair consciousness or the person's movement control, if they occur only during sleep, if they are consistently preceded by an aura, if they are restricted to a certain time of the day (such as within an hour after awakening), or if they occur only when the antiepileptic drugs (AEDs) are reduced or stopped on the advice of a doctor. A letter from the person's doctor confirming the presence and consistency of these features is often required. If this driver's license is later revoked because of a breakthrough seizure caused by extenuating circumstances (reduction of medication on a doctor's advice or unusual stress after a loved one died), the driver can appeal the decision.

EMPLOYMENT AND MILITARY SERVICE FOR PEOPLE WITH EPILEPSY

A productive and satisfying work life can enhance a person's happiness and general satisfaction. Work provides economic security, a higher quality of life, and self-esteem. Most people with epilepsy are capable of productive and gratifying employment, but they may still face discrimination in the job market: stigmas and misconceptions associated with epilepsy do exist, as well as unfounded fears about legal and medical liability. There are laws, however, to prevent discrimination. These laws have improved employment opportunities for people with epilepsy and other disabilities.

Protection Against Job Discrimination

The Americans with Disabilities Act (ADA) makes discrimination based on any disability illegal in employment, in state and local government activities, in public and private transportation, in public accommodations, and in telecommunications. Epilepsy is a disability, but not all people with epilepsy are protected by the ADA. The Act is applicable only if epilepsy substantially limits one or more major life activities (for example, caring for oneself, sleeping, working, or reproducing). If the disorder is fully controlled by medication, epilepsy is only considered a disability if there are associated disorders or significant side effects of medication.

Although the courts often take a conservative approach to claims, people with epilepsy can appeal for inclusion within the ADA based on:

- Seizures; not only in terms of absolute severity and frequency, but also the uncertainty and unpredictability of when seizures will occur
- Medication side effects
- When neither seizures nor side effects alone qualify, the combination can be a substantial disability
- Inability to drive or safely use other forms of transportation
- High rates of unemployment

Title I of the ADA provides that people with disabilities cannot be excluded from employment unless they are unable to perform the essential requirements of the job. An employer may *not* discriminate in recruitment, hiring or promotion, compensation, assignment, sick leave, or fringe benefits. Specifically, the ADA lays out several requirements for hiring, work arrangements, and other aspects of employment.

Criteria for Employment

People with epilepsy or other disabilities must be both qualified and able to perform the *essential* job functions, possibly with some change in the work environment or procedures (that is, a "reasonable accommodation"). The ADA does not require employers to change the fundamental duties of jobs to meet the needs of individuals with disabilities.

Reasonable Accommodations

The ADA requires that covered employers make reasonable accommodations for people with disabilities unless the employer can show that the individual poses a direct threat to the health and safety of others or that the accommodation would impose an "undue burden" on the employer. *Reasonable accommodation* is defined as "any change in the work environment or in the way things are customarily done that enables an individual with a disability to enjoy equal employment opportunities."

A broad range of reasonable accommodations could apply to people with epilepsy. Examples include extended time to take an entrance examination; redistributing *nonessential* or marginal job functions, such as driving, to other employees; temporary changes in job responsibilities or time required to perform certain tasks while someone is adjusting to new medications or to changes in an existing drug regimen; installing carpet on a concrete floor; or allowing an employee to take an extended break after a seizure.

The Application and Interview

The ADA makes it illegal for an employer to require individuals to disclose their disability on an application. An application can, however, ask questions about the applicant's ability to perform essential job duties.

Applicants with epilepsy may choose not to disclose that they have the disorder if it is under good control. However, seizures that interfere with consciousness or control of movement are potentially dangerous if the person drives, works with dangerous equipment or in a dangerous setting, or has a position (such as a ski lift operator or lifeguard) with responsibility for the safety of others.

The ADA also prohibits employers from asking any interview question that would require individuals to reveal their disability. The employer may ask about the applicant's ability to perform both essential and marginal job-related functions, but these questions cannot be phrased in terms of disability. For example, a flower shop owner who needs a delivery person can ask whether the applicant has a driver's license, which is essential for the job.

Medical Examinations

Before offering a job, employers are not allowed to conduct any type of medical examination. *After* a conditional offer of employment, the ADA allows employers to require medical examinations of employees if it's routine for all employees in that particular job. If a disability such as epilepsy is disclosed during the medical interviews and examination, it is confidential (except for first aid and safety personnel) and cannot be used to refuse employment if essential job functions can be performed.

Testing for Illegal Drugs

Employers can test for illegal drugs during any stage of the application process or during employment if all employees are required to take a drug test as part of company policy. The employer cannot use the results of a drug test to discriminate against a disabled person taking prescribed medication.

Explaining Seizures to Coworkers

A person with epilepsy whose seizures are not well controlled should prepare for the possibility that a seizure may occur at work. The preparation will depend on the type and frequency of seizures. As a whole, it's often recommended that a person discuss his seizures with his supervisor and coworkers. These are the people who will first see the seizure if it happens at work and will be called on to administer first aid if necessary. Depending on factors like the person's work environment, his relationships with coworkers, and the nature of his seizures, a person with epilepsy may choose to tell only a few people in his work environment or may opt to tell everyone. It's important, though, not to only tell one coworker, since that coworker may be out of the office when a seizure occurs.

It is often a good idea to review first aid measures in a group setting, so that a number of people know what to expect if a seizure occurs, and how to handle it. The explanation should be reassuring. First aid cards, video, and other educational materials can help.

Vocational Rehabilitation: Job Training and Placement Services

Vocational rehabilitation services can help those who have never held a job (or those who have been out of the work force) train for and get employment that meets their individual needs. This rehabilitation provides specialized training in developing skills, confidence, and strategies to help make up for problems and enhance a person's chances for employment.

The Rehabilitation Act of 1973 provides employment rights for people with disabilities. Vocational rehabilitation services address a range of needs that *may* include, but are not limited to:

- *Diagnostic evaluation* to assess any disability and determine eligibility
- *Counseling* to set goals, make choices, determine job-skill training needed
- *Psychological, physical, or occupational therapies*
- *Training* to teach job skills, compensatory strategies, job search strategies, interviewing skills and job coaching, resumé writing, and legal rights
- *Referral* to training programs
- *Transportation*
- *Job placement* in the competitive work force, in supported community employment or in sheltered workshops, or in the home
- *Post-employment services* to help employees keep their jobs

Military Service

The United States armed services (Army, Navy, Air Force, Marines, Coast Guard, and state National Guard) require that members be available for duty 24 hours a day and have no condition that could impair their performance under adverse conditions. Because sleep deprivation and lack of medication are considered adverse conditions and can cause seizures in people with epilepsy, there are strict regulations regarding the enlistment of people with epilepsy. Individuals with active epilepsy requiring medication are excluded from combat duty.

ROMANTIC RELATIONSHIPS AND MARRIAGE

People whose seizures are well controlled or infrequent should have no serious problems dating or developing and maintaining a stable, intimate relationship. Uncontrolled seizures do make dating and romantic relationships difficult, though certainly not impossible. All people with epilepsy face several of the same important questions: Do I tell the person I'm dating that I have epilepsy? When should I tell him or her? How much should I tell?

There is no reason to rush the disclosure of epilepsy. Unless the seizures are so frequent that one might occur on the first date, it is best to wait until the ice is broken and until trust and openness have developed in a relationship. When the discussion happens, it should be done face to face, not over the telephone or by e-mail. The way that the disorder is presented—say, comfortably and knowledgeably, without fear—is often how the other person will see it. Honesty is important, both about the facts of the disease and how it affects the person's life. The person with epilepsy should allow the other person to react to what he or she has heard. The person with epilepsy has already had time to adjust to the disorder, but the friend needs time to think and to ask questions.

Perhaps most importantly, epilepsy should not be the sole focus of the conversation. After bringing up the topic and answering questions, it's time to move on to other subjects. Like everyone else, a person with epilepsy isn't defined by a single aspect of his life, but by many traits and attributes; epilepsy should not become any person's defining feature.

As is the case even when no epilepsy is involved, some prospective partners may say no to the first date or the second date, and others may break up the relationship after an extended period. People are rejected because of physical characteristics, personality traits, social beliefs, and other reasons. Epilepsy may contribute to the reasons for rejection by some people, and it conversely may be seen as "attractive" to others who have a need to nurture or care for someone. A healthy relationship is most likely to develop when the other person is attracted to the individual's personal qualities and is able to put epilepsy in its rightful place as a medical issue.

SEX LIFE

Most people with epilepsy have normal sex lives and can enjoy all the sexual feelings and pleasures that others enjoy. Seizures during sexual activity are very rare.

Sexual dysfunction—the inability to experience sexual feelings and arousal or to perform sexual activities—is a common problem in the general population and occurs at higher rates in people with epilepsy. Sexual dysfunction can include decreased libido (a lower level of interest in sexual activity), the failure of a man to achieve an erection (impotence), or the inability of a man or woman to achieve an orgasm (anorgasmia). AEDs that induce liver enzymes can cause or aggravate sexual dysfunction. These drugs include carbamazepine, phenobarbital, phenytoin, oxcarbazepine, primidone, and topiramate. By lowering testosterone levels, these drugs can contribute to decreased libido and impotence in men. The effect of these AEDs on women's sexual function has not been adequately studied. Sleep disorders, depression, and drugs used to treat depression can also impair sexual function.

If sexual dysfunction is a problem, a physician or counselor can often be helpful. Drugs used to treat erectile dysfunction (impotence)—Viagra (sildenafil) and Cialis (tadalafil)—appear to be safe for epilepsy patients and do not interact with AEDs.

PREGNANCY AND CHILD REARING

Women with epilepsy face special challenges: effects of their menstrual cycle on seizures (catamenial epilepsy), interactions of AEDs and hormone contraception, and concerns about effects of epilepsy or AEDs on their pregnancies and unborn children. Most women with epilepsy need to continue on their AEDs during pregnancy. Table 21.1 highlights three important principles for all women with epilepsy regarding pregnancy.

Contraception

Women and men today have access to a number of different types of contraception, and while all are safe for people with epilepsy, some will be less effective if used while on antiepileptic medications. The main contraceptive methods are barriers, hormonal therapies, and intrauterine devices (IUDs). Barrier methods—such as condoms and diaphragm caps—are not affected by AEDs. Similarly, most IUDs are not affected by AEDs, although AEDs may affect IUDs that release progesterone into the womb by lowering the amount of progesterone.

Hormonal contraceptives such as the standard combination birth control pill (estrogen and progesterone), the mini pill (progesterone only), progesterone injections (Depo-Provera), progesterone implants (Implanon), and the patch (estrogen and progestin, a form of progesterone) can be made less effective by

---

TABLE 21.1: PREGNANCY FOR WOMEN WITH EPILEPSY (WWE): BASIC PRINCIPLES

1. The large majority of WWE have healthy pregnancies and babies, although they are at increased risk.

2. Any WWE with childbearing potential should discuss pregnancy issues with her physician prior to getting pregnant.

3. No WWE should stop or reduce antiepileptic drug(s) without talking with her physician.

enzyme-inducing AEDs. This can make pregnancy more likely. It's uncertain whether the interaction of enzyme-inducing AEDs and the estrogen/progesterone levels released by vaginal rings (NuvaRing) over a 21-day period lessens the effectiveness of that particular method. As a result, until better data is available, vaginal rings should not be considered reliable for women on these medications. The morning-after pill is a very concentrated form of the birth control pill (levonorgestrel), and may be affected as well. So if a woman is taking an enzyme-inducing AED and wants to use a morning-after pill, she should take one of these pills immediately and another one 12 hours later, for full effectiveness (Table 21.2).

Fertility

Epilepsy, its treatments, and associated disorders may affect fertility and reproduction in both men and women (and overall, men and women with epilepsy have fewer children than people in the general population). Men with epilepsy may have slightly reduced fertility, because hormonal changes and reduced sperm production can occur in men who take enzyme-inducing AEDs. Women with epilepsy have higher rates of infertility than women in the general population. Valproic acid, an AED, can cause polycystic ovary syndrome in women, which affects fertility. This syndrome is characterized by high levels of testosterone in a person's blood, increased hair growth (hirsutism), multiple ovarian cysts,

TABLE 21.2: INTERACTION OF AEDS AND CONTRACEPTION

Drugs that may reduce the effectiveness of hormonal contraception	Drugs that do not reduce the effectiveness of hormonal contraception
Carbamazepine	Benzodiazepines
Oxcarbazepine*	Gabapentin
Eslicarbazepine*	Lamotrigine**
Perampanel	Levetiracetam
Phenobarbital	Pregabalin
Phenytoin	Tiagabine
Primidone	Valproic acid
Rufinamide	Vigabatrin
Topiramate*	Zonisamide

* Effects on hormonal contraceptives occur at higher dosages.

** Lamotrigine levels can be reduced by hormones.

irregular menstruation, and lack of ovulation. Many affected women are also obese.

Planning Before Pregnancy

Although many women with epilepsy successfully get pregnant and have children, there are risks associated with pregnancy for women with the disorder, and steps should be taken to reduce these risks before the pregnancy begins. The specific risks are discussed in the following subsections, but no matter the risk, the first step for a woman with epilepsy who is planning to get pregnant is to make sure she's openly working with her obstetrician and her neurologist to maximize seizure control and thus increase the chances for a healthy pregnancy and baby. The vast majority of women with epilepsy have healthy babies.

Taking vitamins before and during pregnancy may help reduce the risks of malformations in the baby, both for women with epilepsy and without. Folate (folic acid) is the most important vitamin, at doses of 1 to 2 mg/d. Women with a history of birth defects in their family, in a previous pregnancy, or who take valproic acid should take 2 to 4 mg/d. Women with epilepsy who may become pregnant should consider taking a high-potency multivitamin pill.

Risk of Epilepsy in the Baby

Children whose parents have epilepsy have a slightly higher risk of developing epilepsy. The lifetime risk of developing epilepsy in the general population is approximately 3 percent. If a child's father has epilepsy and mother does not, the risk of that child developing epilepsy is only slightly higher than 3 percent. If the mother has epilepsy and the father does not, the risk is somewhat higher but still under 5 percent. If both parents have epilepsy, the risk is a bit higher. The highest risk overall is in children of women with generalized epilepsy.

There's no reason for a couple in which one or even both partners have epilepsy to decide to forgo having children because of fear that the children will have epilepsy. The risk of epilepsy is low, many children outgrow epilepsy, and in most cases of epilepsy the seizures are controlled with a single drug.

Birth Defects and Antiepileptic Drugs

Completely healthy women have a 1 to 2 percent chance of having a baby with a major birth defect. The chance increases to 2 to 6 percent in most women with epilepsy who take a single AED. The main cause of the increased risk appears to be the AED, but genetic factors may contribute as well. As with most complications related to epilepsy, the issue isn't entirely black and white. For example, not all AEDs increase the risk, and AEDs taken by the mother shortly before conception and during the first three months of pregnancy are the most likely to cause congenital birth defects in the fetus. Although some of the congenital defects are minor, in a small percentage of fetuses, AED exposure during the first trimester can cause major birth defects such as cleft lip and cleft palate (a gap in the middle of the lip or palate) and structural defects of the heart, brain, urinary, or other systems. These defects are serious but often the child can live normally after surgery or other treatments. AEDs taken by the father pose no known risk to the fetus.

This means that women with epilepsy are faced with a difficult decision: AEDs taken during pregnancy pose risks for the baby, but most women need to continue taking them, since seizures can be dangerous to both the mother and the baby (and to others if the woman drives). In deciding how to manage seizures while trying to get pregnant, a woman should talk to her doctor about the specific medication that she's taking. The safest AEDs to take during pregnancy include carbamazepine, gabapentin, lamotrigine, levetiracetam, oxcarbazepine, and zonisamide. The lowest effective dose of a single drug and controlling seizures during pregnancy may help minimize any potential risks. Valproic acid is the AED associated with the highest risk of major birth defects and developmental delays in children who were exposed during their mother's pregnancy. Polytherapy (taking more than one AED at a time) and high-dose therapy are more dangerous to the fetus than single-AED therapy or low-dose therapy.

Pregnant women who are taking AEDs are encouraged to contact the Antiepileptic Drug Pregnancy Registry (888-233-2334 or www.aedpregnancyregistry.org), either for the latest AED/pregnancy information or to enroll in their study, and thus help future mothers with epilepsy. Communication with the registry is confidential.

Care During Pregnancy

Regular medical care is essential for all pregnant women. For most women, this simply means visits with an obstetrician to monitor the pregnancy and identify common problems before they become serious. For women with epilepsy, however, visits to both an obstetrician and a neurologist are crucial. This is because of the added risk of complications during pregnancy and the potential for problems with seizure control.

Effects of Pregnancy on Seizure Control

Of women with epilepsy who become pregnant, one-fifth experience an increase in seizure frequency, one-fifth a reduction in that frequency, and more than half have no change. AED blood levels need to be monitored frequently, since they usually decline during pregnancy, even if the drugs are taken as prescribed. The reason for this is because during pregnancy, a woman's body changes in ways that include decreased protein binding, increased metabolism, and increased blood volume and weight gain. As a result, doctors often check blood levels monthly during pregnancy. It is especially important during these months that a woman take her medication as prescribed. If nausea and vomiting become a problem, the doctor should be informed immediately, since the absorption of AEDs can be seriously affected. Finally, seizure activity or seizure freedom during one pregnancy does not necessarily predict what will happen during subsequent pregnancies.

Effects of a Woman's Seizures on the Baby

Absence, myoclonic, simple partial, and complex partial seizures during pregnancy pose no direct danger to the baby. Tonic–clonic seizures can occasionally be dangerous for the developing baby, but usually cause no problems.

Breastfeeding

Breastfeeding is recommended for most women with epilepsy because breast milk confers benefits to the baby, including protection against infection. However, the benefits of breastfeeding (growth factors, resistance to infection) must be weighed against the risks when the mother takes AEDs (exposing the child to AEDs, although he or she was exposed during development). This should be discussed with the obstetrician, pediatrician, and neurologist because some AEDs are found in breast milk in high concentrations.

PARENTHOOD

Caring for a baby or child means loss of freedom and personal time as well as added responsibility. People with well-controlled epilepsy should face no added restrictions when it comes to caring for their children, but they need to consider that significant sleep deprivation may lead to a recurrence of their seizures. Those with ongoing seizures that impair consciousness or control of movement must take special precautions when caring for a baby or a young child. The precautions depend on the child's age and other circumstances.

The large majority of people with epilepsy are able to parent their children exactly as people without epilepsy do. In thinking of your child's future, assuming his epilepsy is well controlled, there's no reason to imagine that he won't be able to have a job, a marriage, and children, as well as all of the fulfillments and frustrations that mark life for his peers.

22

GETTING INFORMATION AND GETTING INVOLVED: EPILEPSY RESOURCES

Information and support are the key tools that help all people with epilepsy and their families understand the disorder, put it in perspective, and move forward with their lives after the medical diagnosis. Luckily, the epilepsy community is large: You will quickly discover that there are many local and national organizations offering a diverse array of resources and working toward varied goals. We encourage you to get involved! Getting involved in the epilepsy community can help you connect with others and perhaps transform your fears into friendships. You can make a difference by helping others and by supporting research and new therapies to help stop seizures and side effects.

GETTING INFORMATION

The Internet can be a confusing and very scary place when you're researching any medical condition. It's potentially a rich source of reliable information, but it's also filled with unreliable material that can scare, misinform, or mislead you. Reliable websites are those with easily discoverable credible sources or that are associated with reputable organizations (such as a medical center; reliable physician; and national, state, or government foundation).

Reliable Sources of Information

The Epilepsy Foundation

The Epilepsy Foundation (EF) is the U.S. national foundation whose mission is to stop seizures and SUDEP, find a cure, and overcome the challenges created by epilepsy. It's a great first stop on your journey for information and support. The EF has a comprehensive website (http://www.epilepsy.com) and a toll-free 24/7 helpline and information number (800-332-1000; for Spanish, 866-748-8006). The staff can provide information and referrals but does not provide specific medical advice or services.

Epilepsy.com offers basic and advanced information on epilepsy and available therapies, online communities, and tools. Their "epilepsy 101" series provides an overview of epilepsy and seizures, as well as the available therapies. Their online community hosts a broad range of discussion threads, blogs, and chats, including stories and commentary about living with epilepsy. Their clinical trial listings offer a comprehensive source for locating all clinical trials ongoing in epilepsy. The site also includes information on seizure preparedness, first aid, and needs of special populations (such as women, children, teens, etc.), and provides a seizure diary and medical management tools to help individuals and caregivers manage their seizures and medications. "My epilepsy diary" is a tool they provide to help track seizures and other factors related to epilepsy care (www.epilepsy.com/get-help/my-epilepsy-diary).

The Foundation works to increase awareness of epilepsy and to build online and offline communities to provide support, mentoring, and the exchange of knowledge and experience about living with epilepsy. The Foundation also serves as the leading advocate on behalf of people with epilepsy with respect to access to care, public health, and other national and state policy priorities. These include medical research, improved quality of medical care, better access to insurance, financial assistance for the disabled, and employment and rehabilitation programs.

EF's state and local affiliates, located across the country, are independently organized groups bound to the national organization and sharing its goals and outlook. The national EF office works with its affiliates to provide local services as well as educational, research, legislative, and other programs. Many of the affiliates offer professionally staffed counseling programs or peer support groups for people with epilepsy or their parents. Counseling sessions may cover such issues as adjusting to/living with epilepsy and parenting a child with epilepsy. As a parent, you may be particularly interested in your affiliate's School Alert program, aimed at improving the school environment for children with epilepsy. Through this program, information about epilepsy is made available to schools and teachers in the form of videotapes, manuals, pamphlets, and in-person presentations. Many affiliates also offer summer camp experiences—often combined with epilepsy education—for children with epilepsy. Local affiliates may even provide job counseling, job clubs, and employer outreach services to improve opportunities for those with epilepsy. The programs offered by the affiliates vary depending on local need and support. Look for the "find us in your area" section of the EF website, or call their toll-free number to find a local chapter.

Community Resources

State Department of Education: Your state's department of education oversees education for all children in the state and can provide information about special education programs and services available to your child. This office can also determine if your child is receiving the needed services to which she is entitled.

Each school district also has a board of education that sets local policies and coordinates special education and other programs.

Your state's Office of Vocational Education for Handicapped Students: this is the place to turn for information about programs for children with disabilities.

Protection and Advocacy Offices for Individuals with Disabilities: this is another resource for information about your state's available services for people with disabilities, which may include education, recreational activities, respite programs, housing programs, and legal representation.

Developmental Disabilities Agency: Your state's developmental disabilities agency allocates federal funds to nonprofit private and public organizations to assist people with developmental disabilities. Some of the services include medical care, information, social services, protection, social activities, group homes, and advocacy.

Comprehensive Epilepsy Centers

A comprehensive epilepsy center specializes in the treatment of epilepsy and is staffed by neurologists with additional training in epilepsy care (epileptologists), as well as neurosurgeons, neuropsychologists, specialized nurses/nurse practitioners, social workers, and dietitians with expertise in epilepsy. This multidisciplinary team works together to find comprehensive treatment options for each patient. There are many comprehensive epilepsy centers across the country; however, not all of them offer the same range of treatment options. If you are looking for a specialized service such as epilepsy surgery or the ketogenic diet, ask the centers if they offer these options and how much experience they have in that treatment field. Compare and contrast centers to see which offers the right fit for you and your family. Most comprehensive epilepsy centers employ multiple epileptologists, allowing you to choose a physician who best shares your mission, goals, and treatment outlook. Comprehensive epilepsy centers are also excellent resources when it comes to finding trustworthy information about epilepsy. To find a list of comprehensive epilepsy centers and their services, visit the EF or the National Association of Epilepsy Centers (www.naec-epilepsy.org/find.htm).

GETTING INVOLVED: RESEARCH, FUNDING, AND MOVING TOWARD A CURE

More than 600,000 Americans have uncontrolled epilepsy, yet epilepsy research remains underfunded. The largest source of funding is government grants, but more money is badly needed. Small groups and individuals, like you, can help by raising money, by contributing, and by writing to government officials and strongly encouraging their support of epilepsy research. More funding allows for more research, and research is critical to finding a cure for epilepsy. Community action and the support of the organizations listed in this section are needed to drive forward epilepsy research to solve the problems of uncontrolled seizures, epilepsy, and SUDEP.

Citizens United for Epilepsy Research (www.cureepilepsy.org)

Citizens United for Epilepsy Research (CURE) is a national organization focused on supporting research and other initiatives for epilepsy. Their goal is to identify and fund cutting-edge research, challenging scientists worldwide to collaborate and innovate in pursuit of this goal. CURE funds seed grants to help young and established investigators explore new areas and collect the data necessary to apply for further funding by the National Institutes for Health (NIH).

Finding a Cure for Epilepsy and Seizures (http://faces.med.nyu.edu)

This nonprofit is affiliated with the NYU Epilepsy Center, and its mission is to improve the quality of life for all people affected by epilepsy. They aim to do this through research, clinical programs, education, and awareness. Most research efforts are focused at NYU, although Finding a Cure for Epilepsy and Seizures (FACES) also partners with many other national and international researchers in collaborative efforts. Through FACES, individual families and patients can ask medical questions, get medical advice, or request consultations from epileptologists (Ask-a-CEC-Doctor@nyumc.org).

Other Disease or Epilepsy-Related Organizations

Aaron's Ohtahara seeks to foster increased awareness, support, and research for Ohtahara syndrome. sites.google.com/a/ohtahara.org/ohtahara2

Aicardi Syndrome Foundation: promotes research and awareness about Aicardi syndrome. https://aicardisyndromefoundation.org

The American Epilepsy Society (AES): AES promotes research and education for professionals dedicated to the prevention, treatment, and cure of epilepsy. www.aesnet.org

The Danny Did Foundation: This group works to prevent deaths caused by seizures. The foundation does this by advancing awareness of sudden unexpected death in epilepsy (SUDEP) and strengthening the communication on the subject of SUDEP between medical professionals and families afflicted by seizures, and also by mainstreaming seizure detection and prediction devices that may assist in preventing deaths caused by seizures. www.dannydid.org

The Dravet Syndrome Foundation: This group raises funds for research on Dravet syndrome and related epilepsies. It also aims to increase awareness of these extremely serious conditions and provide support to the individuals and families affected by them. www.dravetfoundation.org

Dup15q Alliance: provides family support and promotes awareness, research, and targeted treatments for chromosome 15q11.2-13.1 duplication syndrome. dup15q.org

EF: discussed in the beginning of this section. Their activities include education, advocacy, and research to accelerate ideas into therapies. epilepsy.com

Hope for Hypothalamic Hamartomas: This group provides information and support to hypothalamic hamartoma patients, caregivers, and health care providers, and promotes research toward early detection, improved treatments, living with HH, and finding a cure. http://hopeforhh.org

The International Foundation for CDKL5 Research (IFCR): The IFCR funds research in the area of CDKL5, and raises awareness among medical professionals and the public. They also offer information, support, and resources to families affected by the syndrome. www.cdkl5.com

The LGS (Lennox–Gastaut Syndrome) Foundation: This foundation offers information about Lennox–Gastaut syndrome and raises funds for research, services, and programs for individuals and families living with LGS. www.lgs foundation.org

The National Association of Epilepsy Centers: This nonprofit is the central clearinghouse for finding information about the 190 specialized epilepsy centers in the United States. www.naec-epilepsy.org

The National Institute of Neurological Disorders and Stroke: Conducting and supporting nervous system research are the main activities of this institute. www.ninds.nih.gov

The North American SUDEP Registry (NASR): NASR is dedicated to advancing the understanding and prevention of SUDEP. Any affected families should contact them at: info@sudep-registry.org. http://sudep-registry.org

Phelan-McDermitt Syndrome Foundation: This group supports families, increases awareness of, and facilitates research on this disorder. 22q13.org/j15

Seizure Tracker: Visit this website for online and mobile tools dedicated to tracking, monitoring, and sharing (with doctors and other members of your medical team) seizure activity. www.SeizureTracker.com

The Rasmussen's Encephalitis (RE) Children's Project: This group supports research and aims to increase awareness about RE. The group also supports research about the recovery process following hemispherectomy surgery. www.rechildrens.org

The Tuberous Sclerosis Alliance: Tuberous Sclerosis Complex is a genetic disorder that causes epilepsy and autism, and this alliance is dedicated to discovering a cure for TSC and finding ways to improve the lives of those affected by TSC. www.tsalliance.org

Support for your local, state, and national organizations is critical to the continuation of epilepsy research and finding a cure for epilepsy. There are many ways you and your family can get involved. As mentioned earlier, the first step is to urge elected officials to support the groups mentioned in this chapter, and you may also, depending on your situation, want to make donations yourself. Beyond that, the camaraderie you'll find when you immerse yourself in the epilepsy community—when you volunteer or otherwise work with local groups—can prove invaluable. Whether volunteering at local support events and fundraisers or banding together with other parents to advocate for research or education, you'll be reminded of something important: you are not alone. Epilepsy is a disorder that affects many, many children from all walks of life, almost all of whom go on to lead full and fulfilling lives.

APPENDICES

A | THE BRAIN AND HOW IT WORKS

There are 50 to 100 billion nerve cells in the brain, and normal function requires a fine balance between stimulation (excitation) and dampening (inhibition) of activity in these cells. A seizure can result when this balance is disrupted. For example, a traumatic head injury may injure the brain with a "bruise." The injury or healing process can irritate the brain, leading to inflammation that results in an excess of an excitatory neurotransmitter. Alternatively, a genetic abnormality in a protein may open the gate of an ion channel for too long or result in a deficiency of an inhibitory neurotransmitter. In either case, the problem could lead to a group of cells firing simultaneously in an excessive way and recruiting neighboring cells to join the process. Ultimately, large numbers of cells are abnormally activated in a discharge (storm) of electrical activity at the same time.

Knowing how the brain is structured and functions is helpful in understanding seizures and epilepsy. *Structure* refers to the physical features, while *function* refers to how something works. Structure and function are deeply interconnected yet quite different. A structural disorder of the brain is referred to as *damage*, or a *lesion*. Lesions include a large range of abnormalities that result from trauma, infection, stroke, tumor, genetic, or other disorders. A structural problem can be visible (e.g., stroke damage), microscopic (e.g., scar tissue), or submicroscopic (e.g., a genetic disorder that causes a single amino acid substitution in a protein). Functional disorders impair the brain's ability to carry out normal activities. These disorders can result from structural lesions, interruptions in the supply of nutrients, disruptions of metabolic processes, genetic and other abnormalities of cellular function, and other disorders.

The brain and spinal cord form the central nervous system. The nerve fibers and nerve cells outside these structures are often referred to as the peripheral nervous system or "nerves."

ANATOMY OF THE BRAIN

The human brain is an extraordinarily complex organ that controls life-support functions such as breathing and temperature regulation, primitive survival behaviors such as eating and drinking, and sleep-wake cycles, emotions, sensations, movements, and intellect.

The brain is formed by two main types of cells: neurons and glia. *Neurons* are electrically excitable nerve cells that underlie the neural processes of sensation, movement, emotion, and thought. *Glia* are supportive cells that help maintain a healthy environment for neurons by helping to provide structural support and insulation, regulate energy and oxygen supplies, maintain a balance of neurochemicals, and protect from infection. Normal glia can help prevent seizures and epilepsy, while abnormal glia can contribute to seizures and epilepsy. The cerebral cortex forms the large outer surface of the brain. It features numerous folds that increase the surface area and allow more cerebral cortex to be packed into the skull (Figure AA.1).

FIGURE AA.1: Three views of the brain. (A) Outer surface (side view). (B) Inner surface (cross-sectional view). (C) Lower surface (bottom view).

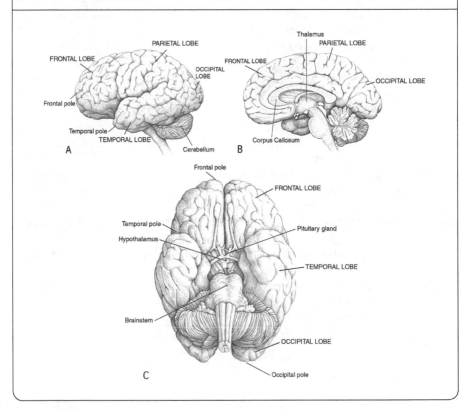

The Cerebrum

The upper brain, or cerebrum, is composed of white matter and gray matter (Figure AA. 2). The gray matter forms the cerebral cortex and consists largely of nerve cells and supportive glia. The nerve cells work like computer chips, analyzing and processing information, and then sending signals through the nerve fibers. The white matter lies beneath the cerebral cortex and is composed of nerve fibers. The nerve fibers act like telephone wires, connecting different areas of the brain, spinal cord, muscles, and glands.

The cerebrum is divided into left and right halves, called *cerebral hemispheres*. These are connected by a large fiber bundle called the *corpus callosum* (see Figure AA.lB). Each cerebral hemisphere contains four lobes: frontal, parietal, occipital, and temporal. Each lobe contains many different areas that have different functions. For example, in almost all right-handed persons, the area that controls speech lies in the left frontal lobe, and the area that controls understanding of spoken and written language lies at the junction of the

FIGURE AA.2: Cross-section of the brain showing the gray matter and the white matter.

left temporal and parietal lobes. Brain functions are carried out by networks of related areas. If one area is injured, other related areas can often compensate. For example, the ability to focus our attention involves multiple brain areas. Problems in certain critical areas of this"attention network"can severely disrupt the ability to stay focused. But disruption or damage in other, less critical areas of the network will cause only a mild and temporary disorder. In contrast, some areas, such as those that control fine hand movements, are localized in only one area, so destruction of that area can lead to permanent impairments. The right half of the brain controls the left side of the body, and vice versa. For example, a stroke in the left cerebral cortex can cause weakness and loss of sensation on the right.

The outer regions of the cerebral cortex contain neocortex, including the sensory, motor, and cognitive ("thinking") areas. The deep, central portions of the frontal and temporal lobes contain the limbic cortex, which controls emotions and memory. Seizures can arise from limbic cortex or neocortex. The functions of the different parts of the brain are summarized in Figure AA.3.

Injury or impaired function of the cerebral cortex can cause seizures. If seizures arise from a specific area of the brain, then the initial symptoms of the seizure often reflect that area's functions. For example, if a seizure starts from the area of the right hemisphere that controls movements in the left thumb, the seizure may begin with jerking movements of the left thumb or hand. The motor cortex of each hemisphere is organized so that groups of muscles are controlled by specific areas. The lowest part of this brain area controls the vocal cords and mouth, the middle part controls the hand and arm, and the upper part controls the leg on the opposite side of the body (Figure AA.4).

The Brainstem and Spinal Cord

The lower part of the brain contains the brainstem, which controls sleep-wake cycles, breathing, and heart rhythm. The upper part of the brainstem contains the thalamus and hypothalamus (see Figs. AA.lB and AA.1C). The spinal cord begins as a continuation of the lower part of the brainstem.

The Thalamus

The thalamus processes sensory information, relaying information about bodily sensations to the cerebral cortex. It is also involved in pain perception and in regulating a person's level of wakefulness (consciousness). The thalamus plays an important role in generalized epilepsies and is involved in generating the generalized spike-and-wave patterns seen on the electroencephalogram (EEG) in these disorders.

FIGURE AA.3: Areas of the human brain responsible for specific functions. (A) Left hemisphere (side view). (B) Right hemisphere (side view). (C) Inner surface (cross-sectional view). The areas in the frontal lobe and the side views of the parietal lobe are not so precisely distributed as the drawings indicate, and the areas overlap in their control of some functions.

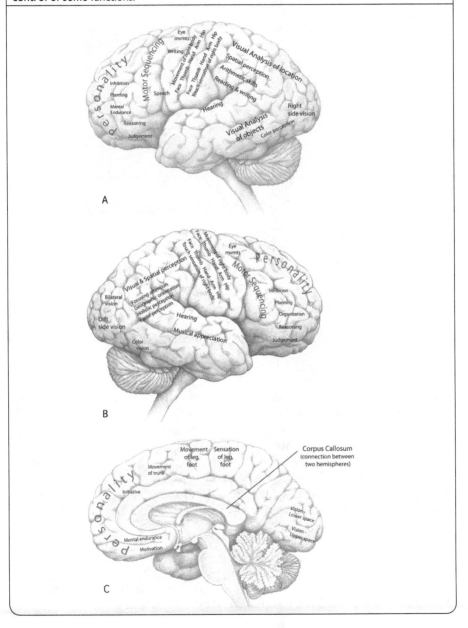

FIGURE AA.4: A cartoon showing the parts of the body whose movements are controlled by various areas of the motor cortex in the right hemisphere.

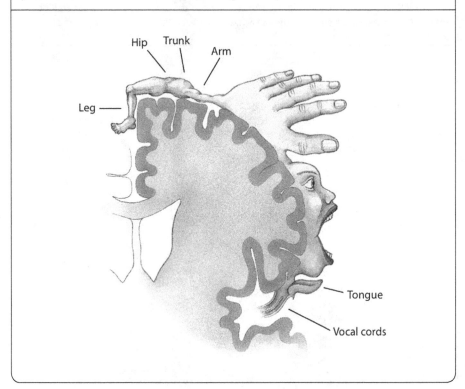

The Hypothalamus

The hypothalamus regulates endocrine (hormone) functions through its control over the pituitary gland. The hormones released by the pituitary gland control the activity of other endocrine glands, such as the ovaries, testicles, thyroid, and adrenal glands. The limbic areas of the temporal lobes influence the hypothalamus, which in turn alters pituitary gland functions. This relationship explains why hormonal functions such as regulation of the menstrual cycle can be disrupted in some women with epilepsy. It also accounts for the increase in seizure frequency at certain times during the menstrual cycle that reflect varying levels of estrogen and progesterone.

The Lower Brainstem

The lower brainstem controls movement and sensation of the face, eye movements, taste, heartbeat, breathing, and other bodily functions.

The Cerebellum

The cerebellum, located behind the brainstem, helps coordinate and "automatize" complex movements. The cerebellum also helps regulate intellectual and behavioral functions.

The Spinal Cord

The spinal cord receives and sends information to the body about senses and movement.

THE CENTRAL AND PERIPHERAL NERVOUS SYSTEMS

Together, the brain and spinal cord are called the *central nervous system*. The nerves in the face, arms, and legs make up the *peripheral nervous system*.

NERVE CELLS OF THE BRAIN

Nerve cells (neurons) are the building blocks of the brain and are composed of three parts: the cell body, axon, and dendrites (Figure AA.5). The cell body contains the enzymes and chemicals that regulate the cell's metabolism and genetic information. The axon is the long portion of a nerve cell that resembles a wire. Axons transmit information locally and great distances in the central and peripheral nervous systems. Most axons are surrounded by myelin, a fatty covering, which insulates them like plastic around telephone wires—preventing "cross-talk" and speeding the transmission of messages.

Axons carry electrical signals from the cell body to the end of the axon, where they lead to the release of chemical messengers (neurotransmitters) that influence other nerve cells. The space between the end of the axon and either a muscle or the dendrite of another neuron is the *synapse*. Dendrites are receivers or antennas. The neurotransmitters released from the axon travel across the synapse to interact with receptors on another nerve cell dendrite, muscle, or gland.

Most nerve cells have thousands of synapses on their dendrites, with specific receptors for the different neurotransmitters to fit, like a key in a lock. A specific key is needed for a specific lock—there are no "master keys" in the brain. These chemical neurotransmitters may increase (excite) or decrease (inhibit) the cell's activity and thereby change the electrical activity and chemical composition of the cell. Thus, both electrical and chemical systems are needed for nerve cells to function and to transmit information.

FIGURE AA.5: A neuron (nerve cell).

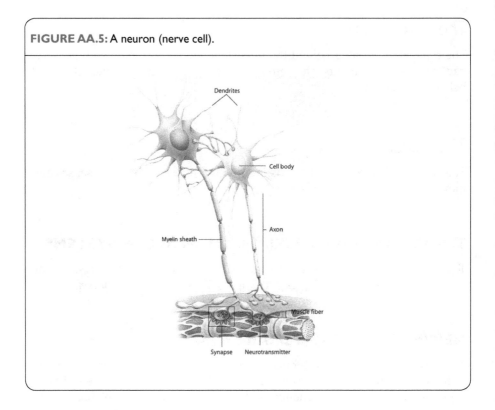

FUNCTION OF THE BRAIN

Brain activity depends on a complex set of interactions involving some of the trillions of connections between brain cells. These connections, or synapses, are the interfaces between nerve cells where electrical and chemical signals are exchanged: electrical activity causes chemical changes and chemical changes produce electrical changes. Healthy brain activity involves a precise harmony of signals and timing. The number of genes involved in brain function reflect the awesome complexity of this process. Of the approximately 20,000 human genes, more than half are expressed in the brain, the highest of any organ.

BRAIN ELECTRICAL ACTIVITY

Input from other nerve cells and influences from other sources, such as hormones, can cause the brains nerve cells to become more negatively or positively charged inside. When nerve cells are very negatively charged, they produce no electrical signals. When they become positively charged, they "fire," like a gun going off. An action potential is generated and travels down the axon to influence other nerve cells.

Nerve cells fire in precise synchrony with each other. This harmony is the basis for the transfer and integration of information. We link the fine detail, colors, shapes, and movements of our visual world by electrical synchronization of different visual areas that perceive each of these elements.

When the synchronization of nerve cells is excessive because it spreads too far or does not stop with normal "braking systems," a seizure can result. In many cases, momentary sparks of increased electrical activity (epilepsy waves) are a marker for a tendency to epilepsy.

NEUROTRANSMITTERS

Neurotransmitters are the chemical messengers that work at the synapse. There are many kinds of neurotransmitters, but individual nerve cells produce only one major type. Some of the neurotransmitters are carried a long distance within the nervous system. Others, however, have local effects; that is, they are produced by and released onto cells that are close to each other. Changes in certain neurotransmitter levels can make seizures more or less likely to occur.

Some of the major brain neurotransmitters can be classified as "excitatory." They stimulate or increase the firing of nerve cells. Others are inhibitory. They shut off or decrease brain electrical activity; that is, they cause nerve cells to stop firing. Simplistically, epilepsy can be considered an imbalance between neurotransmitters that cause nerve cells to fire and those that cause them to stop firing. Either a deficiency of inhibitory neurotransmitters such as GABA or an excess of excitatory neurotransmitters such as glutamate increases the likelihood that a seizure will occur. Many new drugs for epilepsy target the increase of the inhibitory systems or the decrease of excitatory systems.

B | FIRST AID FOR SEIZURES

IF YOUR CHILD HAS A SEIZURE:

- DO NOT PLACE ANYTHING IN YOUR CHILD'S MOUTH. She will not swallow her tongue.
- Do not restrict your child, but keep her safe from harm (away from sharp table edges, a hot stove, etc.).
- If possible, lay the child flat and place her on her side.
- Loosen any scarves or multiple layers of clothes around the face and neck.
- If your child is walking or sitting in a chair, place an arm around the child's shoulder to provide stability and avoid injury.
- Speak to your child in a reassuring tone and explain that everything will be okay.
- Stay with your child at all times.
- Use a watch to time the duration of the seizure.
- If rescue medication has been prescribed, administer as indicated.
- If you are concerned for the child's safety or if the seizure continues despite intervention, call 911.
- After the seizure, your child may be disoriented, so stay with her until she's fully aware, especially if you are near a street, stairs, or other places where there's potential for injury.

WHEN TO CALL 911

Most seizures stop on their own within five minutes, and no professional medical help is needed. Sometimes, though, that's not the case. Call 911 if:

- It's the child's first tonic–clonic seizure*.
- The convulsive seizure is longer than five minutes or occurs as a continuous state.

- There is more than one tonic–clonic seizure, unless this is a known pattern (if so, you and your doctor should have a plan for how many to tolerate before calling 911).

- Your child appears to have sustained a significant injury (such as head trauma or severe back pain) during the seizure.

- Your child has trouble breathing after the seizure has ended.

- For seizures that do not involve convulsive movements (such as prolonged absence seizures or a cluster of complex partial seizures)—911 often need not be called and rescue medications can be given at home. But your doctor should be notified if there is any question.

*For some children, the doctor may consider a tonic–clonic as a likely possibility, and in this case, there may be no need to call 911.

IMPORTANT NUMBERS

Keep all of your important numbers handy. Make sure that any sitters or other adults who watch your child know where these numbers are and when to call them. It can be helpful to bookmark this appendix for sitters, and also to post the numbers on your refrigerator or another easy-to-spot place in your house.

PRIMARY DOCTOR

Name: _____ Phone # _____

HOSPITAL

Name: _____ Phone # _____

PHARMACY

Name: _____ Phone # _____

HEALTH INSURANCE

Insurer: _____ Policy # _____

Phone # _____

C | ANTIEPILEPTIC DRUG INTERACTIONS

EFFECTS OF FREQUENTLY USED ANTIEPILEPTIC DRUGS

Antiepileptic Drug (AED)	AED Levels Effects	Other Interactions
Acetazolamide	<u>Increases</u> Carbamazepine Phenobarbital Phenytoin in children <u>Decreases</u> Primidone	May enhance bone loss when used with enzyme-inducing AEDs
Carbamazepine	<u>Increases</u> Phenobarbital <u>Decreases</u> Clobazam Clonazepam Diazepam Ethosuximide Felbamate Lamotrigine Tiagabine Primidone Topiramate Valproate Zonisamide <u>Variable effect on</u> Phenytoin	Can potentiate neurotoxicity in combination with lamotrigine Additive cardiotoxicity with other Na-channel blockers; potential cardiotoxicity with calcium channel and beta blockers <u>Decreases</u> Oral contraceptive pills (OCPs), theophylline, warfarin

(continued)

EFFECTS OF FREQUENTLY USED ANTIEPILEPTIC DRUGS (*CONTINUED*)

Antiepileptic Drug (AED)	AED Levels Effects	Other Interactions
Clobazam Clonazepam	Increases Primidone Valproic acid	Benzodiazepines increase effects of other CNS depressants Benzodiazepines increase effects of other CNS depressants
Clorazepate	None	
Diazepam	Decreases Phenobarbital Variable effect on Phenytoin	Potentiates narcotic analgesics, barbiturates, phenothiazines, ethanol, antihistamines, MAO inhibitors, sedative-hypnotics, cyclic antidepressants
Eslicarbazepine	Increases Phenytoin Decreases Topiramate	Some interaction with fosphenytoin, phenobarbital, phenytoin
Ethosuximide	Decreases Valproate	
Felbamate	Increases Phenobarbital Phenytoin Valproate Variable, complex Carbamazepine Clobazam	Increases Warfarin Decreases Effectiveness of oral contraceptives Felbamate and phenytoin have been reported to cause toxicity in two cases
Gabapentin	None	
Lacosamide	Decreases Oxcarbazepine	
Lamotrigine	Decreases Clonazepam Valproate Increases Retigabine	Valproate with lamotrigine increases the risk of allergic rash and tremor Carbamazepine and lamotrigine can cause neurotoxicity

(*continued*)

EFFECTS OF FREQUENTLY USED ANTIEPILEPTIC DRUGS (CONTINUED)

Antiepileptic Drug (AED)	AED Levels Effects	Other Interactions
Levetiracetam	None	
Oxcarbazepine	<u>Decreases</u> Lamotrigine Perampanel Topiramate <u>Increases</u> Phenobarbital Phenytoin	<u>Decreases</u> Oral contraceptives
Perampanel	<u>Increases</u> Oxcarbazepine	
Phenobarbital	<u>Decreases</u> Carbamazepine Clonazepam Eslicarbazepine Ethosuximide Felbamate Lacosamide Lamotrigine Oxcarbazepine metabolite Rufinamide Stiripentol Tiagabine Topiramate Valproate Zonisamide <u>Variable effect on</u> Phenytoin	<u>Decreases</u> Theophylline, warfarin, steroids (including oral contraceptives), digoxin, cyclosporine, vitamin K, and tricyclic antidepressants, paroxetine (an SSRI)

(continued)

EFFECTS OF FREQUENTLY USED ANTIEPILEPTIC DRUGS (*CONTINUED*)

Antiepileptic Drug (AED)	AED Levels Effects	Other Interactions
Phenytoin	Decreases Carbamazepine Clobazam Clonazepam Ethosuximide Felbamate Lamotrigine Oxcarbazepine Primidone Tiagabine Topiramate Valproate Zonisamide Variable effect on Diazepam Phenobarbital	Decreases Amiodarone, estrogens, rifampin, vitamin D, doxycycline, warfarin Decreases Effectiveness of oral contraceptives With dopamine—severe hypotension, possibly cardiac arrest
Primidone	Decreases Carbamazepine Ethosuximide Lacosamide Lamotrigine Oxcarbazepine metabolite Rufinamide Stiripentol Tiagabine Topiramate Valproate Zonisamide Variable effect on Phenytoin	Primidone is metabolized to phenobarbital, so has similar effects Decreases Theophylline, coumarin anticoagulants, steroids (including oral contraceptives), digoxin, cyclosporine, vitamin K, and tricyclic antidepressants, paroxetine (an SSRI)

(*continued*)

EFFECTS OF FREQUENTLY USED ANTIEPILEPTIC DRUGS (CONTINUED)

Antiepileptic Drug (AED)	AED Levels Effects	Other Interactions
Retigabine	Decreases Lamotrigine	
Rufinamide	Decreases Lamotrigine	
Stiripentol	Increases Carbamazepine Clobazam Phenobarbital Phenytoin Primidone Valproic acid	
Tiagabine	None	
Topiramate	Increases Phenytoin Decreases Perampanel	Decreases Estradiol, ethinyl estradiol in contra- ceptives, digoxin
Valproate	Increases Diazepam Ethosuximide Lamotrigine Phenobarbital Phenytoin free radical Decreases Topiramate Variable effects Carbamazepine Ethosuximide Phenytoin	Valproate with lamotrigine increases the risk of allergic rash, tremor, unsteadiness

(continued)

EFFECTS OF FREQUENTLY USED ANTIEPILEPTIC DRUGS (*CONTINUED*)

Antiepileptic Drug (AED)	AED Levels Effects	Other Interactions
Vigabatrin	<u>Decreases</u> Phenytoin Rufinamide	
Zonisamide	None	Concomitant administration of carbonic anhydrase inhibitors such as acetazolamide or topiramate may increase potential for renal stone formation

DRUGS THAT INCREASE THE LEVELS OF ANTIEPILEPTIC DRUGS

Antiepileptic Drug	Drug Type	Specific Drugs
Carbamazepine	Antidepressant	Fluoxetine, fluvoxamine, trazodone
	Antimicrobial	Clarithromycin, erythromycin, fluconazole, isoniazid, ketoconazole, metronidazole
	Antipsychotic	Risperidone, quetiapine
	Miscellaneous	Cimetidine, danazol, diltiazem, omeprazole, verapamil
Clobazam	Antifungal	Ketoconazole
	Miscellaneous	Omeprazole (increases clobazam metabolite)
Ethosuximide	Antimicrobial	Isoniazid
Lamotrigine	Antidepressant	Sertraline
Perampanel	Antifungal	Ketoconazole

(continued)

DRUGS THAT INCREASE THE LEVELS OF ANTIEPILEPTIC DRUGS (CONTINUED)

Antiepileptic Drug	Drug Type	Specific Drugs
Phenytoin	Antidepressant	Fluoxetine, fluvoxamine, imipramine, sertraline, trazodone
	Antimicrobial	Fluconazole, isoniazid, miconazole
	Miscellaneous	Allopurinol, amiodarone, cimetidine, diltiazem, disulfiram, 5-fluorouracil, omeprazole, tacrolimus, tamoxifen, ticlopidine, tolbutamide
Phenobarbital	Analgesic	Dextropropoxyphene
Topiramate	Diuretic	Hydrochlorothiazide
Valproic acid	Antidepressant	Sertraline
	Antimicrobial	Erythromycin, isoniazid
	Miscellaneous	Cimetidine

SELECTED DRUGS WHOSE LEVELS ARE REDUCED BY ENZYME-INDUCTED ANTIEPILEPTIC DRUGS*,**

Analgesics	Acetaminophen, fentanyl, methadone, meperidine, tramadol
Antiasthmatics	Theophylline
Anticancer	Busulfan, cyclophosphamide, etoposide, ifosfamide, imatinib, irinotecan, methotrexate, misonidazole, nitrosourea, paclitaxel, procarbazine, tamoxifen, teniposide, thiotepa, topotecan, vinca alkaloids
Antimicrobials	Albendazole, doxycycline, metronidazole, praziquantel, rifampicin

(continued)

SELECTED DRUGS WHOSE LEVELS ARE REDUCED BY ENZYME-INDUCTED ANTIEPILEPTIC DRUGS*,** (*CONTINUED*)

Cardiovascular	Alprenolol, amiodarone, apixaban, atorvastatin, dicumarol, digoxin, diltiazem, disopyramide, felodipine, isradipine, lovastatin, metoprolol, mexiletine, nifedipine, nimodipine, nisoldipine, propranolol, quinidine, simvastatin, talinolol, timolol, verapamil, warfarin
Immunosuppressants	Cyclosporine, everolimus, sirolimus, tacrolimus
Psychotropic drugs	Amitriptyline, aripiprazole, benzodiazepine, bupropion, citalopram, chlorpromazine, clomipramine, clozapine, desipramine, doxepin, haloperidol, imipramine, mirtazepine, nefazodone, nortriptyline, olanzapine, paroxetine, quetiapine, sertraline, risperidone, trazodone, ziprasidone
Steroids	Cortisol, dexamethasone, hydrocortisone, methylprednisolone, prednisone, prednisolone, contraceptive steroids
Thyroid	Thyroxin (usually an effect on protein binding with normal function and levels of T4 and T3)

*This drug list is not complete

**Enzyme-inducing antiepileptic drugs include (1) strong inducers: carbamazepine, phenytoin, phenobarbital, primidone; and (2) weak-modest inducers: eslicarbazepine, felbamate, oxcarbazepine, rufinamide, topiramate (≥ 200 mg/d), and perampanel (≥ 8 mg/d)*

SELECTED OVER-THE-COUNTER DRUGS AND FOODS THAT CAN AFFECT SEIZURE CONTROL OR DRUG SIDE EFFECTS

Drug/Food	Effect	Common Products*
Acetaminophen	May decrease level of lamotrigine in the blood	Alka-Seltzer
		Drixoral
		Excedrin
		Midol
		Robitussin
		Sudafed
		TheraFlu
		Tylenol

(continued)

SELECTED OVER-THE-COUNTER DRUGS AND FOODS THAT CAN AFFECT SEIZURE CONTROL OR DRUG SIDE EFFECTS (CONTINUED)

Drug/Food	Effect	Common Products*
Aspirin or other salicylates**	May decrease total level of phenytoin in the blood but increase free level (effects variable) May increase levels of valproate in the blood, causing adverse side effects	Alka-Seltzer Anacin Bayer Aspirin Bufferin Excedrin
Diphenhydramine	Can lower seizure threshold (minimum conditions necessary to produce a seizure)	Alka-Seltzer PM Pain Reliever and Sleep Aid Benadryl Goody's PM Powder Nytol Sominex Tylenol PM
Grapefruit juice	<u>Increases</u> level of carbamazepine in the blood, causing side effects	

* These are not all-inclusive lists. Refer to ingredient lists when determining whether a product may affect seizure control or contribute to side effects of drugs.

** Low to moderate doses of aspirin (less than 1500 mg/d) are generally very safe for people who take antiepileptic drugs. Higher doses should only be taken after discussion with a doctor, especially if phenytoin or valproate are used. Aspirin-free versions of some products listed are available.

INFORMATION ABOUT YOUR CHILD FOR SCHOOL NURSE AND SCHOOL STAFF

CONTACT INFORMATION

Student's Name: _____ School Year: _____ Date of Birth: _____

School: _____ Grade: _____ Classroom: _____

Parent/Guardian Name: _____ Tel. (H): _____ (W): _____ (C): _____

Other Emergency Contact: _____ Tel. (H): _____ (W): _____ (C): _____

Child's Neurologist: _____ Tel: _____ Location: _____

Child's Primary Care Dr.: _____ Tel: _____ Location: _____

Significant medical history or conditions:

SEIZURE INFORMATION

1. When was your child diagnosed with seizures or epilepsy?_____

2. Seizure type(s):

Seizure Type	Length	Frequency	Description

3. What might trigger a seizure in your child?_____

4. Are there any warnings and/or behavior changes before the seizure occurs?
   YES   NO
   If YES, please explain: _____

5. When was your child's last seizure? _____

6. Has there been any recent change in your child's seizure patterns? YES   NO
   If YES, please explain: _____

7. How does your child react after a seizure is over? _____

8. How do other illnesses affect your child's seizure control? _____

BASIC FIRST AID: Care and Comfort Measures

9. What basic first aid procedures should be taken when your child has a seizure in school?

_____

_____

_____

_____

_____

Basic Seizure First Aid:
✓ Stay calm & track time
✓ Keep child safe
✓ Do not restrain
✓ Do not put anything in mouth
✓ Stay with child until fully conscious
✓ Record seizure in log
For tonic–clonic (grand mal) seizure:
✓ Protect head
✓ Keep airway open/watch breathing
✓ Turn child on side

10. Will your child need to leave the classroom after a seizure? YES   NO
If YES, what process would you recommend for returning your child to classroom

_____

SEIZURE EMERGENCIES

11. What constitutes an emergency for your child? (Please describe; answer may require consultation with treating physician and school nurse.)

_____

_____

_____

12. Has child ever been hospitalized for continuous seizures? YES NO
If YES, please explain:

_____

_____

_____

_____

A seizure is generally considered an emergency when:
✓ A convulsive (tonic–clonic) seizure lasts longer than 5 minutes
✓ Student has repeated seizures without regaining consciousness
✓ Student has a first-time seizure
✓ Student is injured or diabetic
✓ Student has breathing difficulties
✓ Student has a seizure in water

SEIZURE MEDICATION AND TREATMENT INFORMATION

13. What medication(s) does your child take?

Medication	Date Started	Dosage	Frequency and Time of Day Taken	Possible Side Effects

14. What emergency/rescue medications are prescribed for your child?

Medication	Dosage	Administration Instructions (Timing* & Method**)	What to Do After Administration:

* After 2nd or 3rd seizure, for cluster of seizures, etc._____

** Orally, under tongue, rectally, etc.

15. What medication(s) will your child need to take during school hours? _____
16. Should any of these medications be administered in a special way?   YES   NO
    If YES, please explain: _____
17. Should any particular reaction be watched for?   YES   NO
    If YES, please explain: _____
18. What should be done when your child misses a dose? _____
19. Should the school have backup medication available to give your child for missed dose?   YES   NO
20. Do you wish to be called before backup medication is given for a missed dose?
21. Does your child have a vagus nerve stimulator?   YES   NO
    If YES, please describe instructions for appropriate magnet use: _____

SPECIAL CONSIDERATIONS & PRECAUTIONS

22. Check all that apply and describe any considerations or precautions that should be taken

    ❑ General health: _____
    ❑ Physical functioning: _____
    ❑ Physical education (gym)/sports: _____
    ❑ Learning: _____
    ❑ Recess: _____
    ❑ Behavior: _____
    ❑ Field trips: _____
    ❑ Mood/coping: _____
    ❑ Bus transportation: _____
    ❑ Other: _____

GENERAL COMMUNICATION ISSUES

23. What is the best way for us to communicate with you about your child's seizure(s)? _____

24. Can this information be shared with classroom teacher(s) and other appropriate school personnel?   YES   NO

    Parent/Guardian
    Signature: _____ Date: _____

Reprinted by permission from the Epilepsy Foundation. Special thanks to Patty Shafer who helped create this.

E | SEIZURE ACTION PLAN FOR STUDENTS

THE INFORMATION BELOW SHOULD ASSIST YOU IF A SEIZURE OCCURS DURING SCHOOL HOURS.

Student's Name: _____ Date of Birth: _____

Parent/Guardian: _____ Phone: _____

Treating Physician: _____ Phone: _____

Significant medical history: _____ Cell: _____

SEIZURE INFORMATION

Seizure Type	Length	Frequency	Description

Seizure triggers or warning signs: _____

Student's reaction to seizure: _____

BASIC FIRST AID: CARE & COMFORT: *(PLEASE DESCRIBE BASIC FIRST AID PROCEDURES)*

Does student need to leave the classroom after a seizure?   YES   NO

   If YES, describe process for returning student to classroom_____

EMERGENCY RESPONSE

A "seizure emergency" for this student is defined as:

SEIZURE EMERGENCY PROTOCOL:
(CHECK ALL THAT APPLY AND CLARIFY BELOW)

❏ Contact school nurse at _____
_____

❏ Call 911 for transport to _____
❏ Notify parent or emergency contact
❏ Notify doctor
❏ Administer emergency medications as indicated below
❏ Other _____
_____
_____

TREATMENT PROTOCOL DURING SCHOOL HOURS

(Include daily and emergency medications)

Basic Seizure First Aid:

✓ Stay calm & track time
✓ Keep child safe
✓ Do not restrain
✓ Do not put anything in mouth
✓ Stay with child until fully conscious
✓ Record seizure in log

For tonic–clonic (grand mal) seizure:

✓ Protect head
✓ Keep airway open/watch breathing
✓ Turn child on side

A seizure is generally considered an emergency when:

✓ A convulsive (tonic–clonic) seizure lasts more than 5 minutes
✓ Repeated seizures without regaining awareness
✓ Student has a first-time seizure
✓ Student is injured or diabetic
✓ Student has breathing difficulties
✓ Student has a seizure in water

Daily Medication	Dosage & Time of Day Given	Common Side Effects & Special Instructions

Emergency/Rescue Medication
_____

Does student have a **vagus nerve stimulator (VNS)**? YES   NO
If YES, describe magnet use _____

SPECIAL CONSIDERATIONS & SAFETY PRECAUTIONS:

(regarding school activities, sports, trips, etc.)

Physician Signature: _____ Date: _____
Parent Signature: _____ Date: _____

Reprinted by permission from the Epilepsy Foundation. Special thanks to Patty Shafer who helped create this.

INDEX

ABOUT THE AUTHORS

Orrin Devinsky, MD, is a professor of neurology, neurosurgery, and psychiatry at the NYU School of Medicine, and director of the NYU Comprehensive Epilepsy Centers and the Saint Barnabas Institute of Neurology and Neurosurgery (INN). He has published widely in epilepsy, with more than 250 articles and chapters and more than 20 books and monographs. He is currently on the board of the National Epilepsy Foundation. He is coeditor of epilepsy.com, and the journals *Epilepsy and Behavior* and *Reviews in Neurological Diseases*.

Erin Conway, MS, RN, CPNP, is a pediatric nurse practitioner at the NYU Comprehensive Epilepsy Center.

Courtney Schnabel Glick, MS, RD, CDN, is a registered dietitian at the NYU Comprehensive Epilepsy Center.